Malignant Tumors of the Skull Base

Editors

ORIN BLOCH
FRANCO DEMONTE

NEUROSURGERY
CLINICS OF NORTH AMERICA

www.neurosurgery.theclinics.com

Consulting Editors
ANDREW T. PARSA
PAUL C. McCORMICK

January 2013 • Volume 24 • Number 1

ELSEVIER

1600 John F. Kennedy Blvd. ● Suite 1800 ● Philadelphia, PA 19103-2899

http://www.theclinics.com

NEUROSURGERY CLINICS OF NORTH AMERICA Volume 24, Number 1
January 2013 ISSN 1042-3680, ISBN-13: 978-1-4557-7123-3

Editor: Jessica McCool

Neurosurgery Clinics of North America (ISSN 1042-3680) is published quarterly by Elsevier Inc., 360 Park Avenue South, New York, NY 10010-1710. Months of issue are January, April, July, and October. Business and Editorial Offices: 1600 John F. Kennedy Blvd., Suite 1800, Philadelphia, PA 19103-2899. Customer Service Office: 11830 Westline Industrial Drive, St. Louis, MO 63146. Periodicals postage paid at New York, NY, and additional mailing offices. Subscription prices are $360.00 per year (US individuals), $551.00 per year (US institutions), $393.00 per year (Canadian individuals), $674.00 per year (Canadian institutions), $502.00 per year (international individuals), $674.00 per year (international institutions), $177.00 per year (US students), and $243.00 per year (international students). International air speed delivery is included in all *Clinics* subscription prices. All prices are subject to change without notice. **POSTMASTER:** Send address changes to *Neurosurgery Clinics of North America*, Elsevier Periodicals Customer Service, 11830 Westline Industrial Drive, St. Louis, MO 63146. **Customer Service: 1-800-654-2452 (US and Canada). From outside the US and Canada, call: 1-314-453-7041. Fax: 1-314-453-5170. E-mail: JournalsCustomerService-usa@elsevier.com (for print support) and journalsonlinesupport-usa@elsevier.com (for online support).**

Reprints. For copies of 100 or more, of articles in this publication, please contact the Commercial Reprints Department, Elsevier Inc., 360 Park Avenue South, New York, NY 10010-1710. Tel. (212) 633-3812; Fax: (212) 462-1935; E-mail: reprints@elsevier.com.

Neurosurgery Clinics of North America is covered in *MEDLINE/PubMed (Index Medicus), EMBASE/Excerpta Medica, and Current Contents/Clinical Medicine (CC/CM)*.

Printed and bound by CPI Group (UK) Ltd, Croydon, CR0 4YY
Transferred to digital print 2012

Cover image from the American Association for Cancer Research: Vredenburgh JJ, Desjardins A, Herndon JE, et al. Bevacizumab plus irinotecan in recurrent glioblastoma multiforme. J Clin Oncol 2007;25(30):4722–9; with permission for print use only.

Contributors

CONSULTING EDITORS

ANDREW T. PARSA, MD, PhD
Associate Professor, Principal Investigator, Brain Tumor Research Center, Reza and Georgianna Khatib Endowed Chair in Skull Base Tumor Surgery, Department of Neurological Surgery, University of California, San Francisco, San Francisco, California

PAUL C. McCORMICK, MD, MPH, FACS
Herbert & Linda Gallen Professor of Neurological Surgery, Department of Neurological Surgery, Columbia University Medical Center, New York, New York

GUEST EDITORS

ORIN BLOCH, MD
Department of Neurological Surgery, University of California, San Francisco, San Francisco, California

FRANCO DEMONTE, MD, FRCSC, FACS
Professor, Department of Head and Neck Surgery; Mary Beth Pawelek Chair in Neurosurgery, Professor and Vice Chair, Department of Neurosurgery, Adjunct Professor, Baylor College of Medicine, The University of Texas MD Anderson Cancer Center, Houston, Texas

AUTHORS

MANISH K. AGHI, MD, PhD
Department of Neurological Surgery; Center for Minimally Invasive Skull Base Surgery, Assistant Professor of Neurosurgery, University of California, San Francisco, San Francisco, California

IGOR J. BARANI, MD
Assistant Professor, Department of Radiation Oncology, University of California, San Francisco, San Francisco, California

DIANA BELL, MD
Assistant Professor, Department of Pathology, University of Texas MD Anderson Cancer Center, Houston, Texas

MARK H. BILSKY, MD, FACS
Attending, Department of Neurosurgery, Memorial Sloan-Kettering Cancer Center, New York, New York

ORIN BLOCH, MD
Department of Neurological Surgery, University of California, San Francisco, San Francisco, California

FRANCO DEMONTE, MD, FRCSC, FACS
Professor, Department of Head and Neck Surgery; Mary Beth Pawelek Chair in Neurosurgery, Professor and Vice Chair, Department of Neurosurgery, Adjunct Professor, Baylor College of Medicine, The University of Texas MD Anderson Cancer Center, Houston, Texas

IVAN H. EL-SAYED, MD
Center for Minimally Invasive Skull Base Surgery; Department of Otolaryngology–Head and Neck Surgery, University of California, San Francisco, San Francisco, California

FRED GENTILI, MD, MSc, FRCSC
Division of Neurosurgery, Toronto General
Hospital, University Health Network, Toronto,
Ontario, Canada

PAUL W. GIDLEY, MD
Professor, Otology-Neurotology, Department
of Head and Neck Surgery, The University of
Texas MD Anderson Cancer Center, Houston,
Texas

**PATRIC J. GULLANE, CM, MB, FRCSC,
FACS, Hon FRACS, Hon FRCS, Hon FRCSI**
Professor and Chair, Department of
Otolaryngology-Head and Neck Surgery,
Toronto General Hospital, University Health
Network, Toronto, Ontario, Canada

STEPHAN K. HAERLE, MD
Department of Otolaryngology-Head and
Neck Surgery, Toronto General Hospital,
University Health Network, Toronto, Ontario,
Canada

MATTHEW M. HANASONO, MD
Associate Professor, Department of Plastic
Surgery, The University of Texas MD Anderson
Cancer Center, Houston, Texas

EHAB Y. HANNA, MD
Professor and Vice Chair, Department of Head
and Neck Surgery; Professor, Department of
Neurosurgery, The University of Texas MD
Anderson Cancer Center, Houston, Texas

THERESA M. HOFSTEDE, BSc, DDS
Assistant Professor, Section of Dental
Oncology, Department of Head and Neck
Surgery, The University of Texas MD Anderson
Cancer Center, Houston, Texas

MICHAEL E. IVAN, MD
Department of Neurological Surgery; Center for
Minimally Invasive Skull Base Surgery,
University of California, San Francisco,
San Francisco, California

ARMAN JAHANGIRI, BS
Department of Neurological Surgery; Center for
Minimally Invasive Skull Base Surgery,
University of California, San Francisco,
San Francisco, California

BRIAN JIAN, MD, PhD
Department of Neurological Surgery; Center for
Minimally Invasive Skull Base Surgery,
University of California, San Francisco,
San Francisco, California

JULIAN JOHNSON, MD
Resident Physician, Department of Radiation
Oncology, University of California, San
Francisco, San Francisco, California

DENNIS KRAUS, MD, FACS
Director, Head and Neck Oncology, North
Shore-Long Island Jewish Cancer Institute,
New York, New York

MICHAEL E. KUPFERMAN, MD
Assistant Professor, Department of Head and
Neck Surgery, The University of Texas MD
Anderson Cancer Center, Houston, Texas

ILYA LAUFER, MD, MS
Assistant Attending, Department of
Neurosurgery, Memorial Sloan-Kettering
Cancer Center, New York, New York

JOSHUA MARCUS, MD
Resident, Department of Neurosurgery,
Memorial Sloan-Kettering Cancer Center;
Department of Neurosurgery, Weill Medical
College of Cornell University, New York,
New York

BABAK MEHRARA, MD
Associate Attending, Department of Surgery,
Memorial Sloan-Kettering Cancer Center,
New York, New York

LIANE MILLER, BS
Department of Neurological Surgery; Center for
Minimally Invasive Skull Base Surgery,
University of California, San Francisco,
San Francisco, California

**JAMES PAUL O'NEILL, MB, MRCSI, MBA,
MD, MMSc, ORL-HNS**
Department of Head and Neck Surgery,
Memorial Sloan-Kettering Cancer Center,
New York, New York

THOMAS J. OW, MD, MS
Fellow, Department of Head and Neck Surgery,
The University of Texas MD Anderson Cancer
Center, Houston, Texas

ANDREW T. PARSA, MD, PhD
Department of Neurological Surgery, University of California, San Francisco, San Francisco, California

BHUVANESH SINGH, MD, PhD
Attending, Department of Surgery, Memorial Sloan-Kettering Cancer Center, New York, New York

IAN J. WITTERICK, MD, MSc, FRCSC
Department of Otolaryngology-Head and Neck Surgery, Toronto General Hospital, University Health Network, Toronto, Ontario, Canada

CHRISTIAN ZWEIFEL, MD
Division of Neurosurgery, Toronto General Hospital, University Health Network, Toronto, Ontario, Canada

ANDREW T PARSA, MD, PHD
Department of Neurological Surgery, University of California, San Francisco, San Francisco, California

BHUVANESH SINGH, MD, PHD
Attending, Department of Surgery, Memorial Sloan-Kettering Cancer Center, New York, New York

IAN J. WITTERICK, MD, MSc, FRCSC
Department of Otolaryngology-Head and Neck Surgery, Toronto General Hospital, University Health Network, Toronto, Ontario, Canada

CHRISTIAN ZWEIFEL, MD
Division of Neurosurgery, Toronto General Hospital, University Health Network, Toronto, Ontario, Canada

Contents

disease. Multidisciplinary surgical and medical oncologic approaches, including ablation and reconstruction, have enhanced the survival outcome over the past few decades.

Esthesioneuroblastoma is a rare malignant neoplasm in the olfactory region of the nasal cavity and anterior skull base. Diagnosis and staging require anatomic imaging and careful pathologic assessment. Standard treatment is anterior craniofacial resection with postoperative irradiation. The role for chemotherapy is not defined, but is generally for the most advanced cases and used in the neoadjuvant setting and/or postoperatively with irradiation. Prognosis is favorable; however, metastasis rates remain relatively high. Regional and distant metastasis portends a poor outcome. Intensity-modulated radiation treatment and endoscopic surgery have reduced morbidity, but outcomes with these techniques must be fully evaluated.

Sarcomas of the head, neck, and skull base represent a heterogeneous group of tumors with distinct prognostic features. There have been significant improvements in characterizing these sarcomas using traditional morphologic assessments and more recent immunohistochemical analysis. Surgery is the mainstay of treatment followed by radiation therapy. Treatment modalities have changed in select pediatric sarcomas, for which new chemotherapeutic combinations have improved survival statistics. The high rate of distant failure emphasizes the need for novel systemic and directed molecular therapies. Tumor grade, size, and margin status are key factors in survival.

Chordomas of the skull base are one of the rarest intracranial malignancies that arise from ectopic remnants of embryonal notochod. The proximity of many chordomas to neurovascular structures makes gross total resection difficult, and the tendency for recurrence leads to the routine use of adjuvant postoperative radiation. Several surgical approaches are used ranging from extensive craniotomies to minimally invasive endonasal endoscopic approaches. In this review, the histopathology and epidemiology, imaging characteristics, surgical approaches, adjuvant therapies, prognostic factors, and molecular biology of chordomas are described.

Chondrosarcomas are indolent but invasive chondroid malignancies that can form in the skull base. Standard management of chondrosarcoma involves surgical resection and adjuvant radiation therapy. This review evaluates evidence from the literature to assess the importance of the surgical approach and extent of resection on outcomes for patients with skull base chondrosarcoma. Also evaluated is the ability of the multiple modalities of radiation therapy, such as conventional fractionated radiotherapy, proton beam, and stereotactic radiosurgery, to control tumor growth.

Finally, emerging therapies for the treatment of skull-base chondrosarcoma are discussed.

Temporal Bone Malignancies   97

Paul W. Gidley and Franco DeMonte

Primary temporal bone tumors are rare. Suspicious lesions of the ear canal should be biopsied for diagnosis. Surgical resection to achieve negative margins is the mainstay of treatment. Small tumors can be treated with lateral temporal bone resection. Parotidectomy and neck dissection are added for disease extension and proper staging. Higher staged tumors generally require subtotal temporal bone resection or total temporal bone resection. Adjuvant postoperative radiotherapy has shown improved survival for some patients. Chemotherapy has an emerging role for advanced stage disease. Evaluation and management by a multidisciplinary team are the best approach for patients with these tumors.

Craniofacial Reconstruction Following Oncologic Resection   111

Matthew M. Hanasono and Theresa M. Hofstede

The ability to reliably reconstruct complex and sizable wounds has decreased the morbidity of skull base surgery substantially, preventing major complications and allowing treatment of tumors previously considered inoperable. Addressing facial nerve function with static and dynamic procedures as well as fabrication of craniofacial prostheses to replace delicate facial landmarks has further increased surgeons' ability to restore the appearance and function of the face.

Radiotherapy for Malignant Tumors of the Skull Base   125

Julian Johnson and Igor J. Barani

Malignant tumors of the skull base are a fascinating group of tumors arising via disparate causes leading often to similar presentations. This article explores radiotherapy techniques applied to this group of malignancies, with a focus on providing general overview and guiding readers to primary sources to achieve greater depth. The outcomes and effects of radiation, therapeutic radiation modalities and delivery system are discussed. Equipped with these basic principles, practitioners will have general guidance for rational treatment modality selection for patients with skull base tumors.

NEUROSURGERY CLINICS OF NORTH AMERICA

Preface
Malignant Tumors of the Skull Base

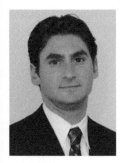

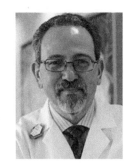

Orin Bloch, MD   Franco DeMonte, MD, FRCSC, FACS
                 Guest Editors

Skull base surgery for the treatment of malignant tumors has undergone substantial evolution over the past 50 years. Although resection of skull base tumors was sporadically attempted in the early part of the 20th century, it was not until the 1960s that interdisciplinary approaches combining expertise from neurosurgery, otolaryngology, and maxillofacial surgery facilitated the development of the field of skull base surgery. During the 1980s and 1990s, significant advancements in surgical and reconstructive techniques made oncologic resections at the skull base possible with acceptable morbidity. Concurrent advancements in medical imaging further improved visualization of skull base anatomy and surgical planning, driving an era of aggressive maximal resections. The last decade has seen the rise of endoscopic technologies and new techniques to approach the skull base. These approaches require validation as appropriate options in the management of sinonasal and skull base malignancy. Endoscopic resections need to adhere to the tenets of oncologic surgery, complete surgical resection with microscopically clear margins, to provide the survival advantages gained with craniofacial resection.

Concomitant with the developments in surgery have been improvements in radiation targeting.

The routine use of 3D treatment planning and intensity-modulated radiation therapy has allowed delivery of higher radiation doses to the tumor while minimizing morbidity due to irradiation of normal structures. Similarly, a better understanding of tumor biology has allowed the construction of more complex treatment strategies, which incorporate neoadjuvant, concomitant, or adjuvant chemotherapies. These new strategies have had a significant positive impact on patient survival in select pathologies. The era of personalized targeted therapy is upon us and rapid strides are being made in the identification of specific tumoral targets for novel biologic agents. This is sure to impact our current management paradigms.

In this issue we have compiled articles addressing the diagnosis and management of the most common skull base malignancies. We review the pathology, surgical approaches, and outcomes for each tumor type. In addition, we have included overviews on open and endoscopic approaches to the skull base, as well as techniques for reconstruction. In the modern era, extensive resection of skull base malignancies through a combination of open and minimally invasive approaches can be achieved with acceptable morbidity when appropriate planning and reconstructive techniques are

http://dx.doi.org/10.1016/j.nec.2012.08.012
1042-3680/13/$ – see front matter

neurosurgery.theclinics.com

used. These surgical procedures, when fully incorporated into an individualized multimodal treatment plan, allow for the maximization of patient survival and quality of life.

Orin Bloch, MD
Department of Neurological Surgery
University of California, San Francisco
505 Parnassus Avenue, M-779
San Francisco, CA 94143-0112, USA

Franco DeMonte, MD, FRCSC, FACS
Department of Neurosurgery–Unit 442
The University of Texas MD
Anderson Cancer Center
1515 Holcombe Blvd
Houston, TX 77030, USA

E-mail addresses:
blochog@neurosurg.ucsf.edu (O. Bloch)
fdemonte@mdanderson.org (F. DeMonte)

Management Considerations for Malignant Tumors of the Skull Base

Franco DeMonte, MD, FRCSC

KEYWORDS

• Skull-base tumor • Microsurgery • Radiation • Complications

KEY POINTS

- Tumor pathology and behavior should drive the approach to skull-base malignancies and must be considered before undertaking surgical resection.
- A multidisciplinary team with expertise in surgical and oncologic management as well as reconstruction and rehabilitation should assess each case individually to develop an appropriate tailored approach for the patient.
- Induction therapy before resection can be used to minimize the extent and morbidity of surgery and improve tumor control in selected cases.
- Complex craniofacial reconstruction should be used to decrease morbidity associated with surgical complications (cerebrospinal fluid leak, infection) and cosmetic deformity.
- Quality of life after craniofacial resection is as dependent on psychosocial adjustment to disease and deformity as it is on neurologic outcome.

PATIENT POPULATION

Over a 20-year period, 473 patients (32 of whom were children or adolescents) with skull-base malignancies were operated on by the author in the setting of a tertiary-care comprehensive cancer center. A multidisciplinary team experienced in the assessment and treatment of skull-base malignancy evaluated all patients preoperatively. The anterior skull base was most commonly affected in the adult population, whereas the middle skull base was the most commonly affected site in children. **Fig. 1** depicts the skull-base region affected and whether the patient was a child or an adult. In adults the most commonly encountered abnormalities were squamous cell carcinoma, adenoid cystic carcinoma, chondrosarcoma, olfactory neuroblastoma, and adenocarcinoma. Sarcomas constituted 38% of the malignancies in adults but 75% of the malignancies in children. The most common

abnormalities by site are listed in **Box 1**. **Fig. 1** shows the breakdown between sarcoma and non-sarcoma pathology at each skull-base site. The middle skull base is relatively the most likely site for a sarcoma.

MANAGEMENT PARADIGMS

The foundation of all management decisions rests on a representative biopsy of the tumor, properly identified and diagnosed by experts in surgical pathology with experience in head and neck malignancy, neural tumors, and sarcoma pathology. Inaccurate diagnoses can lead to both undertreatment and overtreatment, with their attendant toxicity and morbidity. Cohen and colleagues[1] discuss an example of the problems encountered with misdiagnosis with respect to sinonasal olfactory neuroblastoma. In a series of 12 consecutive patients referred with the biopsy-proven diagnosis

Department of Neurosurgery, Unit 442, The University of Texas MD Anderson Cancer Center, 1515 Holcombe Boulevard, Houston, TX 77030, USA
E-mail address: fdemonte@mdanderson.org

Neurosurg Clin N Am 24 (2013) 1–10
http://dx.doi.org/10.1016/j.nec.2012.08.003
1042-3680/13/$ – see front matter © 2013 Elsevier Inc. All rights reserved.

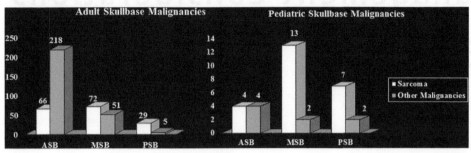

Fig. 1. Skull-base region affected, relative age of patient, and nature of malignancy (sarcoma vs nonsarcoma). ASB, anterior skull base; MSB, middle skull base; PSB, posterior skull base. (*Courtesy of* Department of Neurosurgery, The University of Texas M.D. Anderson Cancer Center; with permission.)

of olfactory neuroblastoma only 2 patients, on review by an expert pathologist, did in fact harbor this tumor. Revised diagnoses included pituitary adenoma (3 patients), neuroendocrine carcinoma (3), sinonasal undifferentiated carcinoma (2), and melanoma (2). These revised diagnoses led to significant alterations in the initially proposed treatment plan in 8 of 10 patients, including the recommendation of observation alone in the 3 patients with pituitary adenomas, 1 of whom had been rendered blind by radiation necrosis of his optic nerves (the tumor had been aggressively treated as an olfactory neuroblastoma).

With the correct pathologic diagnosis in hand, each patient should be evaluated by members of a multidisciplinary group including medical and radiation oncology, dental oncology, head and neck surgery, neurosurgery, and plastic surgery.

Box 1
Skull-base site and most common malignancies encountered

Anterior skull base

   Squamous cell carcinoma

   Sarcoma

   Olfactory neuroblastoma

   Adenocarcinoma

   Adenoid cystic carcinoma

   Sinonasal undifferentiated carcinoma

Middle skull base

   Sarcoma

   Squamous cell carcinoma

   Adenoid cystic carcinoma

Posterior skull base

   Chordoma

   Basal cell carcinoma

Additional consultations with speech pathology, audiology, otology, and ophthalmology may be necessary. In this setting the combined expertise of each individual is brought to bear on the patient's problem and leads to the construction of the optimal management plan for each patient. The skull-base neurosurgeon's main contribution is the determination, along with the rest of the surgical team, as to whether the tumor can be completely encompassed by a surgical resection that carries acceptable morbidity. With experience the neurosurgeon can also identify which tumor pathologic/biological factors make resection (with its attendant morbidity) worthwhile, or those instances whereby a complete tumor resection may not be necessary (usually to maintain function). Along with the determination of tumor resectability, the availability and nature of adjuvant therapies and the medical and psychic candidacy of the patient for surgery/treatment is taken into consideration.

The simplest management paradigm, surgical excision alone, may be applicable to certain low-grade malignancies such as low-grade chondrosarcomas, low-grade papillary adenocarcinomas, and desmoid tumors.[2] Complete resection can result in cure or long-term remission, although late recurrence can be an issue.

The management paradigm most applicable to the majority of patients with skull-base malignancy is that of surgical extirpation followed by external beam radiation therapy. This approach is generally the recommended treatment for lower-stage squamous cell carcinomas, olfactory neuroblastoma, adenocarcinoma, adenoid cystic carcinoma, and most metastases, and may be used in some patients with low-grade sarcomas.[3–8] Induction chemotherapy may also be used in the context of an organ-sparing (usually orbital-sparing) approach. Data supporting this approach are limited although early studies show promise, with one group of investigators reporting a response rate in excess of 90%.[9] Similarly, investigators from the University of Chicago reported complete histologic response in 5 of 16 patients and a 10-year locoregional and distant control rate exceeding 90%.[10] At the author's institution this is an especially common pathway for patients with squamous cell carcinoma and sinonasal undifferentiated carcinoma. Induction chemotherapy with cisplatin, a taxane, and 5-fluorouracil with or without gemcitabine has been shown to be an effective combination for patients with squamous cell carcinoma.[11,12] In a recent study from M.D. Anderson, patients with advanced sinonasal squamous cell carcinoma were treated with induction chemotherapy with a platinum-based and taxane based regimen.[13] Just over two-thirds of the patients achieved at least a partial response, while 24% had progressive disease and 9% had stable disease. The 2-year survival for patients with at least a partial response or stable disease after induction chemotherapy was 77%, in contrast to only 36% for patients with progressive disease. Similarly, the author's practice, and that of others, has increasingly been to use induction chemotherapy with cisplatin-based programs (usually in combination with etoposide) for sinonasal undifferentiated carcinoma with or without surgical resection, dependent on the response to chemotherapy (**Fig. 2**).[14,15] For certain abnormalities surgical resection may not be a necessary part of the management paradigm. For patients with moderate to poorly differentiated neuroendocrine carcinoma, induction chemotherapy with cisplatin or carboplatin with etoposide frequently results in a complete or substantial response, which may be consolidated with definitive radiotherapy. Long-term survival has been reported with this strategy, but a standard chemoradiation schedule has not been defined.[1,3,16–19] Other abnormalities that fall into this treatment paradigm include lymphoma, Ewing sarcoma, and most pediatric rhabdomyosarcomas and malignant peripheral nerve sheath tumors.

A relatively recent addition to management paradigms has been the planned use of postoperative single-fraction stereotactic radiation boost to areas of either proven or potential microscopic tumor residual. This approach has been most commonly applied in patients with squamous cell carcinoma and adenoid cystic carcinoma in the presence of, or potential presence of, perineural tumor extension (**Fig. 3**). It is too early to judge the usefulness of this modality in disease control and survival, although several patients remain without recurrence more than 3 years after treatment. The author's current management paradigms and applicable malignancies are listed in **Box 2**.

LOW-GRADE AND HIGH-GRADE MALIGNANCIES

As indicated by the preceding discussion, management paradigms clearly differ based on the biological nature of the malignancy being treated. In an early study the author's group evaluated management paradigms based on the categorization of primary skull-base sarcomas into high and low biological aggressiveness (grade). An attempt was made to determine the accuracy of this biological/managerial grading scheme and to identify prognostic indicators for survival and progression-free survival. Such a scheme helps to logically manage the numerous and highly diverse malignant abnormalities encountered. In this study of 64 patients, 31 patients had high-grade sarcomas and 33 patients were categorized as having low-grade sarcomas.[20] Based on the management algorithm, the majority of patients with high-grade sarcomas were radiated (71%) and received chemotherapy (81%). Surgery alone was used in the majority of patients with low-grade sarcomas, although 46% were also radiated and 21% given chemotherapy. Also of note is that based on a philosophy of preservation of function, 40% of patients with low-grade sarcomas had gross residual disease following resection compared with only 16% of patients with high-grade sarcomas. This management resulted in an overall survival at 1, 5, and 10 years of 83%, 66%, and 52% for the patients with high-grade sarcomas and 100%, 85%, and 57% for the patients with low-grade sarcomas, respectively. Progression-free survival at 1, 5, and 10 years was 86%, 56% and 46% for the patients with high-grade sarcomas and 90%, 65% and 0% for the patients with low-grade sarcomas, respectively. These results, especially the 100% recurrence rate at 10 years for patients with low-grade malignancies, indicate the need to reevaluate the management of this patient population. Improved surgical resection, possibly at the expense of function, needs to be considered, although this must be weighed against the expected diminution of quality of life (QOL) of patients. Increasing the use of postoperative radiation and/or chemotherapy also needs to be considered. These questions are as yet unanswered.

OUTCOMES
Oncologic

It was not until the introduction of craniofacial resection that a substantial improvement in long-term disease control was appreciated in patients with malignancies of the paranasal sinuses

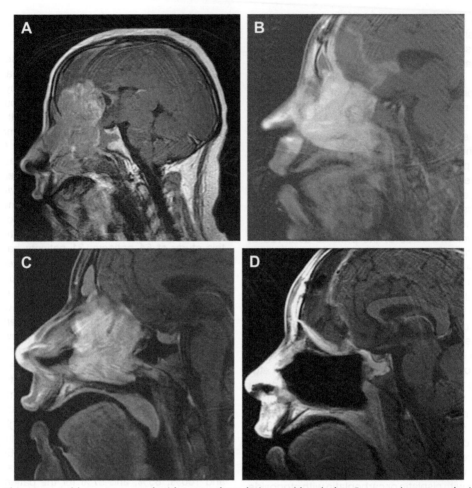

Fig. 2. This 23-year-old man presented with acute obtundation and headache. Computed tomography imaging revealed a large frontal tumor with intracerebral hematoma. Initial sagittal postcontrast T1-weighted magnetic resonance imaging (MRI) (*A*) revealed a large sinonasal tumor with intracerebral extension. The patient was taken to the operating room emergently, and underwent resection of all intracranial tumor and evacuation of hematoma. (*B*) Postoperative sagittal postcontrast T1-weighted MRI. Pathology was consistent with sinonasal undifferentiated carcinoma. He was subsequently treated with 4 cycles of cisplatin and etoposide with partial response evident on the post-chemotherapy sagittal postcontrast T1-weighted MRI (*C*). He then underwent formal anterior craniofacial resection. The postoperative sagittal postcontrast T1-wieghted MRI (*D*) confirmed complete tumor removal. Extensive pathologic analysis could not identify any viable tumor. He was treated post-operatively with intensity-modulated radiation therapy to a dose of 60 Gy in 30 fractions. He is free of disease 3 years later. (*Courtesy of* Department of Neurosurgery, The University of Texas M.D. Anderson Cancer Center; with permission.)

affecting the skull base. Before this, overall 5-year survival did not exceed 30%.[21] Several large modern surgical series currently report survival rates of approximately 50% to 70% at 5 years and 40% to 50% at 10 years.[22–29] McCutcheon and colleagues[30] reported median survivals of 20 months for patients with squamous cell carcinoma, 26 months for adenocarcinoma, and 40 months for olfactory neuroblastoma in the 26 of 76 patients who died during the course of their review. This group reported an overall 63% 2-year nonactuarial survival. Lund and colleagues[26]

identified malignant histology, brain involvement, and orbital involvement as negative predictors of patient outcome. As well as confirming the negative effect of brain invasion on survival, Clayman and colleagues[31] also identified positive histologic margins as predictors of local recurrence and shorter survival. Transdural involvement, however, should not dissuade the consideration of patients for aggressive surgical management. Feiz-Erfan and colleagues[32] were able to achieve a 5-year overall survival of 58% in a group of 28 patients with transdural invasion of malignancy. Gross total

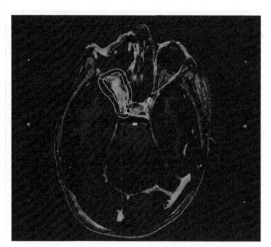

Fig. 3. Axial postcontrast T1-weighted MRI with superimposed radiosurgical treatment plan. This female patient with invasive squamous cell carcinoma of the skin of the right eyebrow had been extensively treated with multiple surgeries and external beam radiation. At recurrence she underwent wide local excision of the tumor with orbitectomy. Residual disease in the cavernous sinus was treated with radiosurgery to a dose of 15 Gy at the 50% isodose line. (*Courtesy of* Department of Neurosurgery, The University of Texas M.D. Anderson Cancer Center; with permission.)

resection with microscopically negative margins was the key positive predictor of overall survival and progression-free survival. In the author's cohort of patients with sarcomas of the skull base, only brain parenchymal involvement was significantly associated with a shorter survival and progression-free survival, although achieving microscopically negative margins, rather than leaving grossly positive margins, had a strong trend toward improved progression-free survival. Overall, this group of patients achieved a 5- and 10-year survival of 75% and 56%.

Malignancy involving the anterolateral skull base is clinically and pathologically distinct from malignancy involving the anterior skull base or the parotid/temporal bone.[30,33,34] These tumors commonly invade the infratemporal fossa and the walls of the maxillary sinus, and frequently present with facial pain and an externally evident mass. There is usually involvement of the maxillary and mandibular divisions of the trigeminal nerve. The most common tumors of this region were sarcomas, followed by squamous cell carcinoma and adenoid cystic carcinoma (**Fig. 4**). With aggressive multimodal therapy the author's group found an overall median survival of 5 years, a 2-year survival of 81%, and a 5-year survival of 53%.[35] Cavernous sinus and internal carotid artery involvement was present in about 20% of the

patients. The overall median survival for patients not requiring cavernous sinus dissection or internal carotid artery resection was twice that of patients undergoing these maneuvers. Statistically significant predictors of decreased overall survival included dural and central nervous system invasion by tumor, presence of high-grade sarcoma, complications of therapy, and age 65 years or older.

Age, however, as in the case of transdural tumor extension, should not exclude the consideration of aggressive surgical resection in patients with skull-base malignancy. In patients undergoing anterior craniofacial resection the author found no significant difference in disease-specific survival in a cohort of patients with a mean age of 70 years, when compared with a younger cohort (mean age 56 years).[36] The older age group did, however, have a 3-fold greater incidence of systemic complications.

Patients with malignant tumors of the sphenoidal sinus, although accounting for only 1% to 2% of patients with paranasal sinus malignancy, are an especially difficult subgroup to manage effectively. Even in this patient population, aggressive multimodality therapy can result in a 2-year survival rate of 44% for patients with squamous cell carcinoma.[37]

Tumor pathology is an important predictor of outcome in these patients. Five-year overall survival ranges from 89% for olfactory neuroblastoma to 39% for mucosal melanoma.[6,8,38–40] Mucosal melanoma is associated with a particularly poor patient outcome. In the author's series the disease-free survival was only 18.4%.[39] In contradistinction, olfactory neuroblastoma has the best patient outcome, with a 10-year survival rate of 81%. It should be noted, however, that the mean time to recurrence in these patients was around 4.5 years, which mandates careful long-term patient follow-up.[6]

Adenoid cystic carcinoma is a rare tumor with a high recurrence rate. In the author's patient population recurrence was noted in 56.2%. This result is in the context of a 5-year disease-specific survival rate of 70.9%. Many patients remain alive with disease for years, and survival from this disease exceeds that of most other sinonasal malignancies.[7,8,41]

Recent advances in endoscopic instrumentation and surgical technique has created excitement in skull-base surgery. Initially applied to the repair of cerebrospinal fluids leaks, endoscopic approaches to benign and malignant tumors have been increasingly reported. One major concern has been the paradigm shift from en bloc resection to one of piecemeal resection of sinonasal

---

Box 2
Management paradigms and applicable malignancies

Surgical resection
  Low-grade chondrosarcoma
  Basal cell carcinoma
  Desmoid fibromatosis
  Some other low-grade sarcomas and low-grade adenocarcinomas
Surgical resection and postoperative radiation therapy
  Olfactory neuroblastoma
  Adenocarcinoma
  Adenoid cystic carcinoma
  Squamous cell carcinoma
  Most metastases
  Some low-grade sarcomas
Pre- and postoperative chemotherapy, surgical resection, and postoperative radiation therapy
  Squamous cell carcinoma
  High-grade sarcomas
  SNUC and other neuroendocrine carcinomas
  Melanoma
Chemotherapy and radiation therapy
  Lymphoma
  Ewing sarcoma
  Most rhabdomyosarcomas and MPNST
  Some patients with SNUC and other neuroendocrine carcinomas
Chemotherapy, radiation therapy, surgical resection, and stereotactic radiosurgery
  Squamous cell carcinoma ⎫
  Adenoid cystic carcinoma ⎬ especially with perineural extension
  Some high-grade sarcomas, SNUC ⎭

Abbreviations: MPNST, malignant peripheral nerve sheath tumor; SNUC, sinonasal undifferentiated carcinoma.

---

malignancy. In an effort to address this controversy the author's group reviewed its experience with endoscopic resection of sinonasal malignancies with and without the addition of a craniotomy. In this cohort of patients, 93 underwent a purely endoscopic resection of their anterior skull-base malignancy and 27 patients underwent a cranioendoscopic resection.[34] The main difference between the two groups was the significantly higher T stage in patients treated with a cranioendoscopic technique. This difference understood, no significant difference was found in overall survival between the two treatment groups. In the author's opinion, this was a proof of principle that in appropriately selected patients a purely endoscopic approach to tumoral resection can be safely performed without compromising patient survival.

Complications of Treatment

A considerable complication rate accompanies the craniofacial resection of skull-base malignancies. Most surgical series report complication rates of 25% to 60%.[25,29,42–45] The most commonly identified complications in the literature are infectious, with wound infection (especially osteomyelitis) and meningitis predominating.[46] Other commonly reported complications include cerebral spinal fluid leakage, delayed return of neurologic function, and tension pneumocephalus. In a review of 209 patients undergoing anterior craniofacial resection at M.D. Anderson Cancer Center between 1992 and 2008, a 20% complication rate was seen.[47] In contrast to reports in the literature, the cerebrospinal fluid (CSF) leak rate

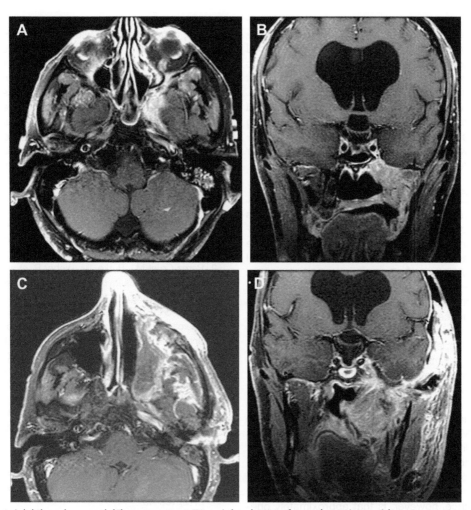

Fig. 4. Axial (*A*) and coronal (*B*) postcontrast T1-weighted MRI of a male patient with a recurrent malignant fibrous histiocytoma of the left infratemporal fossa and anterolateral skull base. He underwent a transfacial and anterolateral skull-base approach with complete tumor removal. Reconstruction with a free anterolateral thigh flap was performed following watertight dural closure. Final pathology was read as pleomorphic sarcoma. Postoperative axial (*C*) and coronal (*D*) postcontrast T1-weighted MRI confirmed complete tumor removal. Chemoradiation is planned. (*Courtesy of* Department of Neurosurgery, The University of Texas M.D. Anderson Cancer Center; with permission.)

and rate of infection were both less than 1%. When appropriate reconstructive choices are made, which in most cases means using a well-vascularized pedicled pericranial flap or a free tissue transfer over a watertight dural closure, the CSF leak rate and the incidence of orbital morbidity are reduced.[48–50] The author's routine use of broad-spectrum antibiotics has resulted in a low rate of wound infection, and there has been no bone flap loss. Delayed return of neurologic function needs to be differentiated from postoperative delirium. The former complication is almost certainly due to excessive frontal lobe retraction, and has been eradicated from this series because of careful patient positioning and

operative technique that emphasizes the use and importance of the operating microscope. The later complication, that of postoperative delirium, occurs in almost 20% of patients older than 70 years and is likely multifactorial in nature, with drug interactions and preexisting pre-clinical dementia being the most likely culprits.[36] Tension pneumocephalus is due to overdrainage of CSF either late in surgery or in the postoperative period. This complication can be seen even if the lumbar drain has been removed. Treatment consists of needle aspiration of the intracranial air, the delivery of 100% oxygen, and intubation or tracheostomy if severe. An epidural blood patch may be necessary. A less acute intracranial hypotension-like syndrome can be associated with persistent headache, usually with a significant postural component, and imaging evidence of poor cerebral expansion. Perturbed CSF dynamics, leading to intracranial hypotension, were the single most common cause of complications in this series. Just over a third of all complications identified were considered to be related to this underlying process. These complications have been eliminated with the cessation of the use of lumbar spinal fluid drainage.

Quality of Life

In a previously reported cohort of 16 patients undergoing anterior craniofacial resection for paranasal sinus malignancy affecting the skull base, the author assessed health-related QOL and functional status of patients.[51] Patient-generated responses to the Functional Assessment of Cancer Therapy questionnaire, including its brain and head and neck subscales, were used to measure QOL, and the Karnofsky Performance Score (KPS) and Functional Independence Measure (FIM) were used to assess patient function.[52,53] Anterior craniofacial resection and other indicated adjunctive therapies for paranasal sinus malignancies rarely affected independence. Ninety-four percent of patients (15 of 16) had KPS of 90 or 100 and 87% of patients had FIM scores higher than 117, which indicates the ability to perform most or all activities of daily living independently. All patients reported a good QOL from a neurologic standpoint, and 94% did so from a head and neck standpoint as well. Of importance, however, is that approximately one-third of the patients reported a poor QOL based on their responses to the FACT (Functional Assessment of Cancer Therapy) general questionnaire. It appears that this diminished QOL is less related to the specifics of the treatment than to the psychosocial changes and adjustments that accompany an illness and its treatment. Several other disclaimers need to be made, notably that a patient's perception of their health and QOL is not necessarily related to objectively assessed functionality; moreover, the health-related QOL in patients with brain injury arising from tumor and treatment must be analyzed with the potential effect of neurocognitive impairment in mind.[54] In these patients a 3-pronged assessment using measures of functionality and performance, cognition, and self-reported QOL is the most telling approach.[55]

SUMMARY

Although great strides have been made in the management of skull-base malignancies, much room for improvement exists. Ideally, improvements in the chemotherapeutic management of these tumors, almost certainly with novel agents, would lessen the need for extensive extirpative surgeries. Improved treatment targeting and radiotherapeutic technologies such as intensity-modulated radiation therapy are reducing the morbidities associated with radiation and will likely become even more refined. Surgery will remain an integral part of the treatment of these malignancies, be it in the current role of ablative surgery, either open or endoscopic, or in future roles of drug/virus/gene delivery.

REFERENCES

1. Cohen ZR, Marmor E, Fuller GN, et al. Misdiagnosis of olfactory neuroblastoma. Neurosurg Focus 2002; 12(5):e3.
2. Perez-Cruet MJ, Burke JM, Weber R, et al. Aggressive fibromatosis involving the cranial base in children. Neurosurgery 1998;43(5):1096–102.
3. Austin JR, Cebrun H, Kershisnik M, et al. Olfactory neuroblastoma and neuroendocrine carcinoma of the anterior skull base: treatment results at the M.D. Anderson Cancer Center. Skull Base Surg 1996;6(1):1–8.
4. Chamoun RB, Suki D, DeMonte F. Surgical management of cranial base metastases. Neurosurgery 2012;70(4):802–9 [discussion: 809–10].
5. DeMonte F. Soft tissue sarcomas of the skull base: time for a new paradigm. Cancer 2007;110(5): 939–40.
6. Diaz EM Jr, Johnigan RH 3rd, Pero C, et al. Olfactory neuroblastoma: the 22-year experience at one comprehensive cancer center. Head Neck 2005; 27(2):138–49.
7. Esmaeli B, Golio D, Kies M, et al. Surgical management of locally advanced adenoid cystic carcinoma of the lacrimal gland. Ophthal Plast Reconstr Surg 2006;22(5):366–70.
8. Lupinetti AD, Roberts DB, Williams MD, et al. Sinonasal adenoid cystic carcinoma: the M. D. Anderson Cancer Center experience. Cancer 2007;110(12): 2726–31.
9. Choi KN, Rotman M, Aziz H, et al. Concomitant infusion of cisplatin and hyperfractionated radiotherapy for locally advanced nasopharyngeal and paranasal sinus tumors. Int J Radiat Oncol Biol Phys 1997;39: 823–9.
10. Lee MM, Vokes EE, Rosen A, et al. Multimodality therapy in advanced paranasal sinus carcinoma: superior long-term results. Cancer J Sci Am 1999;5:219–23.
11. Posner MR, Hershock DM, Blajman CR, et al. Cisplatin and fluorouracil alone or with docetaxel in head and neck cancer. N Engl J Med 2007;357(17): 1705–15.
12. Vermorken JB, Remenar E, Van Herpen C, et al. Cisplatin, fluorouracil, and docetaxel in unresectable

head and neck cancer. N Engl J Med 2007;357(17): 1695–704.

13. Hanna EY, Cardenas AD, DeMonte F, et al. Induction chemotherapy for advanced squamous cell carcinoma of the paranasal sinuses. Arch Otolaryngol Head Neck Surg 2011;137(1):78–81.

14. Diaz EM Jr, Kies MS. Chemotherapy for skull base cancers. Otolaryngol Clin North Am 2001;34(6): 1079–85.

15. Righi PD, Francis F, Aron BS, et al. Sinonasal undifferentiated carcinoma: a 10-year experience. Am J Otolaryngol 1996;17:167–71.

16. Likhacheva A, Rosenthal DI, Hanna E, et al. Sinonasal neuroendocrine carcinoma: impact of differentiation status on response and outcome. Head Neck Oncol 2011;3:32.

17. Mitchell EH, Diaz A, Yilmaz T, et al. Multimodality treatment for sinonasal neuroendocrine carcinoma. Head Neck 2011. http://dx.doi.org/10.1002/hed.21940. [Epub ahead of print].

18. Ordonez NG, Mackay B. Neuroendocrine tumors of the nasal cavity. Pathol Annu 1993;28:77–111.

19. Thornton AF, Varvares M, McIntyre J, et al. Treatment of esthesioneuroblastoma and neuroendocrine carcinoma with combined chemotherapy and proton radiation. Proc Am Soc Clin Oncol 1998;441a.

20. Prabhu SS, Diaz E, Sturgis M, et al. Section on tumors: Mahaley clinical research award: primary sarcomas of the skull base: an analysis of 63 cases. Clin Neurosurg 2004;51:340–2.

21. Sisson GA Sr, Toriumi DM, Atiyah R, et al. Paranasal sinus malignancy: a comprehensive update. Laryngoscope 1989;99(2):143–50.

22. Cantu G, Solero CL, Mariana L, et al. Anterior craniofacial resection for malignant ethmoid tumors—a series of 91 patients. Head Neck 1999;21(3):185–91.

23. Danks RA, Kaye AH, Millar H, et al. Craniofacial resection in the management of paranasal sinus cancer. J Clin Neurosci 1994;1(2):111–7.

24. Ganly I, Patel SG, Singh B, et al. Craniofacial resection for malignant paranasal sinus tumors: report of an International Collaborative Study. Head Neck 2005;27(7):575–84.

25. Janecka IP, Sen C, Sekhar LN, et al. Cranial base surgery: results in 183 patients. Otolaryngol Head Neck Surg 1994;110:539–46.

26. Lund VJ, Howard DJ, Wei WI, et al. Craniofacial resection for tumors of the nasal cavity and paranasal sinuses: a 17-year experience. Head Neck 1998;20(2):97–105.

27. Patel SG, Singh B, Polluri A, et al. Craniofacial surgery for malignant skull base tumors: report of an international collaborative study. Cancer 2003;98(6):1179–87.

28. Shah JP, Kraus DH, Bilsky MH, et al. Craniofacial resection for malignant tumors involving the anterior skull base. Arch Otolaryngol Head Neck Surg 1997; 123(12):1312–7.

29. Sundaresan N, Shah JP. Craniofacial resection for anterior skull base tumors. Head Neck 1988;10(4): 219–24.

30. McCutcheon IE, Blacklock JB, Weber RS, et al. Anterior transcranial (craniofacial) resection of tumors of the paranasal sinuses: surgical technique and results. Neurosurgery 1996;38(3):471–9 [discussion: 479–80].

31. Clayman GL, DeMonte F, Jaffe DM, et al. Outcome and complications of extended cranial-base resection requiring microvascular free-tissue transfer. Arch Otolaryngol Head Neck Surg 1995;121(11): 1253–7.

32. Feiz-Erfan I, Suki D, Hanna E, et al. Prognostic significance of transdural invasion of cranial base malignancies in patients undergoing craniofacial resection. Neurosurgery 2007;61(6):1178–85 [discussion: 1185].

33. Gidley PW, Thompson CR, Roberts DB, et al. The oncology of otology. Laryngoscope 2012;122(2): 393–400.

34. Hanna E, DeMonte F, Ibrahim S, et al. Endoscopic resection of sinonasal cancers with and without craniotomy: oncologic results. Arch Otolaryngol Head Neck Surg 2009;135(12):1219–24.

35. Hentschel SJ, Vora Y, Suki D, et al. Malignant tumors of the anterolateral skull base. Neurosurgery 2010; 66(1):102–12 [discussion: 112].

36. Hentschel SJ, Nader R, Suki D, et al. Craniofacial resections in the elderly: an outcome study. J Neurosurg 2004;101(6):935–43.

37. DeMonte F, Ginsberg LE, Clayman GL, et al. Primary malignant tumors of the sphenoidal sinus. Neurosurgery 2000;46(5):1084–91 [discussion: 1091–92].

38. Backous DD, DeMonte F, El-Naggar A, et al. Craniofacial resection for nonmelanoma skin cancer of the head and neck. Laryngoscope 2005;115(6):931–7.

39. Moreno MA, Roberts DB, Kupferman ME, et al. Mucosal melanoma of the nose and paranasal sinuses, a contemporary experience from the M. D. Anderson Cancer Center. Cancer 2010;116(9):2215–23.

40. Rosenthal DI, Barker JL Jr, El-Naggar AK, et al. Sinonasal malignancies with neuroendocrine differentiation: patterns of failure according to histologic phenotype. Cancer 2004;101(11):2567–73.

41. Williams MD, Al-Zubidi N, Debnam JM, et al. Bone invasion by adenoid cystic carcinoma of the lacrimal gland: preoperative imaging assessment and surgical considerations. Ophthal Plast Reconstr Surg 2010;26(6):403–8.

42. Catalano PJ, Hecht CS, Biller HF, et al. Craniofacial resection. An analysis of 73 cases. Arch Otolaryngol Head Neck Surg 1994;120:1203–8.

43. Dias FL, Sa GM, Sicard MW, et al. Complications of anterior craniofacial resection. Head Neck 1999;21: 12–20.

44. Kraus DH, Shah JP, Arbit E, et al. Complications of craniofacial resection for tumors involving the anterior skull base. Head Neck 1994;16(4):307–12.

45. Richtsmeier WJ, Briggs RJ, Koch WM, et al. Complications and early outcome of anterior craniofacial resection. Arch Otolaryngol Head Neck Surg 1992;118(9):913–7.

46. Ganly I, Patel SG, Singh B, et al. Complications of craniofacial resection for malignant tumors of the skull base: report of an International Collaborative Study. Head Neck 2005;27(6):445–51.

47. Fourney DR, Ogieglo L, DeMonte F. Neoplasms of the paranasal sinuses. In: Winn HR, editor. Youmans neurological surgery, vol.2. Philadelphia: Elsevier; 2011. p. 1610–23.

48. Chang DW, Langstein HN, Gupta A, et al. Reconstructive management of cranial base defects following tumor ablation. Plast Reconstr Surg 2001;107(6):1346–57.

49. DeMonte F, Tabrizi P, Culpepper A, et al. Ophthalmological outcome after orbital entry during anterior and anterolateral skull base surgery. J Neurosurg 2002;97(4):851–6.

50. Hanasono MM, Silva A, Skoracki J, et al. Skull base reconstruction: an updated approach. Plast Reconstr Surg 2011;128(3):675–86.

51. DeMonte F. Functional outcomes in skull base surgery. What is acceptable? Clin Neurosurg 2001;48:340–50.

52. Cella DF, Tulsky DS, Gray G, et al. The functional assessment of cancer therapy (FACT) scale: development and validation of the general version. J Clin Oncol 1993;11:570–9.

53. Weitzner MA, Meyers CA, Gelke CK, et al. The functional assessment of cancer therapy (FACT) scale: development of a brain subscale and revalidation of the FACT-G in the brain tumor population. Cancer 1995;75:1151–61.

54. Meyers C, Geara F, Wong PF, et al. Neurocognitive effects of therapeutic irradiation for base of skull tumors. Int J Radiat Oncol Biol Phys 2000;46(1):51–5.

55. Meyers C. Issues of quality of life in neuro-oncology. Handbook Clin Neurol 1997;23(67):389–409.

Anterior and Anterolateral Resection for Skull Base Malignancies
Techniques and Complication Avoidance

Joshua Marcus, MD[a,c], Ilya Laufer, MD, MS[a],
Babak Mehrara, MD[b], Dennis Kraus, MD[d],
Bhuvanesh Singh, MD, PhD[b], Mark H. Bilsky, MD[a,*]

KEYWORDS

- Anterior craniofacial • Skull base malignancy • Pneumocephalus • Endoscopy

KEY POINTS

- Combined craniofacial resection remains the most effective approach for skull base malignancies, despite the evolution of endonasal endoscopic techniques.
- Meticulous dural reconstruction and skull base repair limit the major complications associated with craniofacial resections.
- Effective management of complications, such as CSF leak and pneumocephalus, limit the morbidity from these operations.

INTRODUCTION

The application of the combined craniofacial approach for skull base malignancies was first described by Ketcham, and colleagues[1] in 1963. Techniques have evolved significantly since the original description, but the basic premise of gross total resection with negative margins remains the goal of therapy. Technical advances in resection and reconstruction, improvements in intensive care management, and triple antibiotic therapy have reduced complications and allowed for the safe removal of anterior cranial base malignancies that involve not only the anterior skull base, but also the orbit, brain, and infratemporal fossa. The evolution of anterior cranial base surgery integrated with

advanced imaging and adjuvant radiation and chemotherapy have shown improved outcomes over the last 2 decades. Gil and colleagues[2] reported a significant improvement in overall survival and disease-specific survival in patients who have undergone surgery since 1996 compared with those who underwent resection from 1973–1996. Of 106 patients operated on before 1996, the 5-year overall survival and disease-specific survival rates were 55% and 57%, respectively, whereas they improved to 66% and 70%, respectively, for the 176 patients in their series who were treated from 1996–2008. Despite advances in surgery, poor prognostic indicators include positive surgical margins, unfavorable tumor histologies (eg, squamous cell carcinoma, melanoma,

[a] Department of Neurosurgery, Memorial Sloan-Kettering Cancer Center, 1275 York Avenue, New York, NY 10065, USA; [b] Department of Surgery, Memorial Sloan-Kettering Cancer Center, New York, NY, USA; [c] Department of Neurosurgery, Weill Medical College of Cornell University, 525 East 68th Street, New York, NY 10065, USA; [d] Head and Neck Oncology, North Shore-Long Island Jewish Cancer Institute, 130 East 77th Street, New York, NY 10075, USA
* Corresponding author. Department of Neurosurgery, Memorial Sloan-Kettering Cancer Center, 1275 York Avenue, New York, NY 10065.
E-mail address: bilskym@mskcc.org

Neurosurg Clin N Am 24 (2013) 11–18
http://dx.doi.org/10.1016/j.nec.2012.08.008
1042-3680/13/$ – see front matter © 2013 Elsevier Inc. All rights reserved.

high-grade sarcoma), intracranial or orbital invasion, and prior radiation therapy.[3–5]

Despite the evolution of purely endonasal endoscopic techniques, the combined craniofacial techniques continue to be the gold standard and principle strategy in treatment of anterior and anterolateral skull base malignancies. The obvious benefits of purely endoscopic techniques include less soft-tissue dissection and avoidance of the morbidity associated with a craniotomy and brain retraction[6]; however, these benefits may be more relevant for benign skull base tumors than for extensive skull base malignancies. Malignant tumors often present significant anatomic constraints to effective endoscopic resection because of involvement of neurovascular structures, optic nerves, and infiltration into the brain, orbit, or infratemporal fossa. Additionally, endoscopic resection obviates not only the ability to achieve en bloc resection for negative margins, but also necessitates dissecting through tumor to identify normal structures. Conversely, the craniofacial approach allows the identification of normal structures first rather than intralesionally dissecting through tumor to identify critical anatomy and normal tissue planes. The ability to separate the nasal cavity from the intradural compartment is limited via an endoscopic approach because of the frequent need to use a nasoseptal flap for reconstruction. The nasal septum often is resected in the treatment of malignancies because of tumor involvement or to achieve negative margins. Finally, clinical series showing improved local control with endoscopic techniques are not comparable with regard to prognostic categories based on tumor histologies. In a report from Eloy and colleagues,[7] local recurrence rates were 5.6% in the endoscopic group compared with 29.2% for the craniofacial cohort, which approached significance ($P = .051$). However, a lack of equipoise was demonstrated, as most patients in the endoscopic group had favorable prognostic histologies (eg, esthesioneuroblastoma, small cell carcinoma) compared with the craniofacial groups with poor prognostic histologies (eg, squamous cell carcinoma, high-grade sarcomas).[7,8] Soler and Smith reviewed published data on endoscopic compared with craniofacial techniques for esthesioneuroblastoma.[9] Short-term control rates seem to be equivalent, but endoscopic techniques are typically reserved for lower-stage tumors.

It is critical that surgeons treating skull base malignancies continue to understand the techniques and reconstructive strategies of combined anterior craniofacial approaches. The integration of endoscopic endonasal dissection is becoming more prevalent but has not currently replaced the need for a combined anterior cranial base approach. This article reviews the nuances of anterior and anterolateral resection of skull base malignancies and complication avoidance and management.

COMBINED ANTERIOR CRANIOFACIAL RESECTION

Imaging

Both magnetic resonance (MR) imaging and computed tomography (CT) scans are helpful in preoperative planning to define the extent of tumor and type of resection required. CT scans are useful for defining the myriad of anatomic variability in bone anatomy, including the size of the frontal sinus and crista galli, location of bony septae, length of the planum sphenoidale, and degree of bone erosion. The MR is important for tumor identification and the relationship to critical structures. The extent of resection and type of reconstruction is determined principally based on MR imaging. Contraindications to surgical resection can be evaluated, including extensive cavernous sinus involvement and involvement of the only sighted eye. However, even high-resolution MR may not provide enough detail to make preoperative decisions regarding periorbital invasion, which may require orbital exenteration or penetration of the skull base dura. Decisions regarding these issues may still require highly skilled intraoperative judgment and extensive informed consent. The propensity for some tumors to present with regional or distant metastases also plays a major role in determining treatment. A screening body scan, such as positron emission tomography or CT, is important for staging before treatment.

Preoperative Biopsy

Definitive preoperative pathologic diagnosis of anterior skull base malignancies is critical to decisions regarding treatment. Most biopsies can be done endoscopically by head and neck surgeons in the office, but occasionally deep lesions undergo biopsy in the operating room. Tumor management is highly dependent on whether the pathology results are benign or malignant and the relative responsiveness to radiation or chemotherapy. Malignant tumors such as lymphoma and rhabdomyosarcoma are treated with chemotherapy either as definitive therapy or as neoadjuvant treatment. Other tumors, such as squamous cell carcinoma, adenoid cystic carcinoma, sarcoma and melanoma are best treated with resection.

Surgery

Preparation

After induction of general anesthesia, the endotracheal tube should be positioned opposite the site of the lateral rhinotomy or the epicenter of the tumor. The eyelids are sutured, but the suture should be placed so that the pupils can be readily examined at surgery. A spinal drain is placed for intermittent drainage throughout the procedure to facilitate brain relaxation and for use in the postoperative period to ensure a water-tight closure. Triple antibiotic therapy (metronidazole ceftazidime, vancomycin) is initiated at the induction of anesthesia. The preparation should take into account all possible facial incisions and the need for a free flap.

SURGICAL TECHNIQUE
Craniotomy and Galeal Pericranial Graft: Smaller and Longer, Respectively

The head is positioned on a foam donut. A bicoronal incision is fashioned between the zygomas over the vertex of the skull starting 1.5 cm anterior the ear after injection of the skin with 1% lidocaine with epinephrine. The skin is incised with a 10 blade taking care to preserve the pericranium, which initially remains attached to the scalp. A hemostat is used to define the plane between the galea and pericranium. The superficial temporary arteries are preserved for possible free flap anastomosis at the end of the operation. A subgaleal dissection of the posterior skin flap is accomplished extending to the posterior parietal bone. The posterior pericranium is incised at this point with the Bovie cautery, and a subperiosteal dissection with a broad periosteal elevator is accomplished to the level of the supraorbital rims and nasion. The galea is then dissected from the anterior scalp flap beginning 1 cm anterior to the incision to facilitate subsequent galeal closure. The galeal-pericranial graft is harvested with a 15 blade, creating a long vascularized graft for skull base reconstruction. This flap is wrapped in bacitracin-soaked gauze and retracted with blunt hooks (**Fig. 1**).

The craniotomy is then turned. A single burr hole is placed in the midline overlying the sagittal sinus or through the frontal sinus approximately 3 cm superior to the nasion and laterally to the middle of the supraorbital rims. Dura is dissected from the underside of the bone, and the craniotomy is performed with a 1-mm matchstick bur. The mucosa of the frontal sinus is exenterated, and the posterior wall of the frontal sinus is removed with a 3-mm matchstick burr. The crista galli is identified extradurally and removed. The remainder of the dissection is intradural.

Dural Resection and Repair

The dura is incised anterior to the crista galli, and the olfactory nerves are sacrificed with bipolar cautery and suction. Intracranial tumor is resected to the level of the skull base. Dural incisions are made laterally and posteriorly with the goal of achieving negative margins. Typically, the dura is incised laterally over the fovea ethmoidales and posteriorly along the anterior planum sphenoidale. Frequently, tumor abuts or invades the dura, requiring more extensive dural resections. Lateral and posterior dural dissection from the skull base is accomplished using a Penfield 4 to create cuffs for dural reconstruction. Dural reconstruction is accomplished using an inlay graft of DuraGen (Integra LifeSciences Corporation, Plainsboro, New Jersey), creating a gasket seal and a bovine pericardial patch graft (DuraGard; Synovis Surgical Innovations, Minnesota) is sutured with a 4–0 nonresorbable continuous suture initiated at the posterior suture line. A tear in the posterior suture line is virtually impossible to repair primarily, but a muscle patch

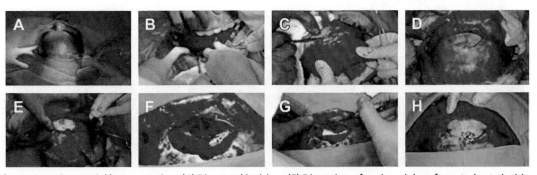

Fig. 1. Anterior cranial base resection. (*A*) Bicoronal incision. (*B*) Dissection of pericranial graft posterior to incision to create long pedicled flap. (*C*) Harvesting pedicled pericranial-galeal pericranial graft. (*D*) Outline of craniotomy flap. (*E*) Bone flap turned. (*F*) Resection of skull base dura. (*G*) Reconstruction with bovine pericardial patch graft. (*H*) Bone flap replaced with epidural drain. (*Adapted from* Bilsky MH, Bentz B, Vitaz T, et al. Craniofacial resection for cranial base malignancies involving the infratemporal fossa. Neurosurgery 2005;57(4):339–47; with permission.)

(temporalis muscle) stitched over the defect can salvage a water-tight dural repair.

Intranasal Dissection

The intranasal dissection is carried out by experienced head and neck surgeons. Traditionally, the nasal approach requires a lateral rhinotomy. When a maxillectomy is required, the lateral rhinotomy incision is extended in the midline to the lip. More recently, endoscopic techniques have been used for the intranasal dissection.

Skull Base Osteotomies

Skull base osteotomies are tailored to the extent of the tumor. Judicious use of spinal fluid drainage often makes placement of brain retractors unnecessary. Gentle retraction with the suction provides excellent exposure. The skull base osteotomies are made with an M8 bur, although many surgeons use thin osteotomes. The drill is preferred over osteotomes because of the improved ability to control the fracture lines. Resection of the tumor is accomplished by working from both intranasal and intracranial orientations. The osteotomies for a standard anterior cranial facial resection are created through the anterior frontal bone, bilateral ethmoid sinuses, and planum sphenoidale.

More extensive bone removal may be required depending on the degree of bone and soft tissue involvement, for example, in a type 3 infratemporal fossa resection (**Fig. 2**).[10–13] This resection is required for patients with malignancies involving the infratemporal fossa, maxillary sinus, orbit and anterior cranial base. A frontotemporal bone flap is created to perform a combined subtemporal-infratemporal fossa and anterior cranial base resection. The anterior cranial base is prepared in the same fashion as a standard anterior cranial base resection. An extradural dissection is extended across the squamous temporal bone and greater wing of the sphenoid in a lateral to medial direction to the level of the foramen rotundum and maxillary division of the trigeminal nerve (V2). Further extradural dissection is extended posteriorly along the greater wing of the sphenoid to create a posterior margin that includes the foramen ovale and mandibular division of the trigeminal nerve (V3). The dura is resected depending on the degree of dural abutment or invasion. Perpendicular osteotomies with the 3-mm matchstick bur are made from the lateral squamous temporal bone to the foramen ovale then extended anteriorly to the foramen rotundum. V2 is sacrificed with vascular clips. The resulting osteotomy is lateral to the carotid artery, cavernous sinus, and superior orbital fissure. Dissection of the pterygoid muscles posterior to the tumor is performed. The skull base osteotomies are extended in a coronal plane anterior to the superior orbital fissure. This osteotomy is extended across the lesser wing of the sphenoid anterior to the optic foramen and the posterior planum sphenoidale. The osteotomy then extends anteriorly to include the contralateral ethmoids and cribriform plate. The orbital contents are cut at the optic foramen. Rarely is the optic nerve resected intradurally because of

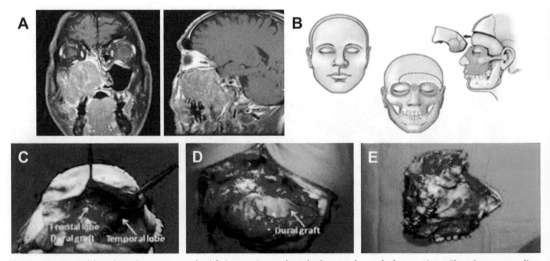

Fig. 2. 53 years old male, who presented with intermittent headaches and nasal obstruction. Chordoma was diagnosed after a biopsy. (*A*) Preoperative MR imaging. (*B*) Schematic representation of the operation. (*C*) Craniotomy with dural resection. (*D*) Dural repair using bovine pericardium. (*E*) Excised tumor. (*Adapted from* Bilsky MH, Bentz B, Vitaz T, et al. Craniofacial resection for cranial base malignancies involving the infratemporal fossa. Neurosurgery 2005;57(4):339–47; with permission.)

the small risk of producing a nasal field deficit in the remaining eye. The tumor is then resected.

In standard skull base reconstruction, after tumor resection, 3 drill holes are placed through the posterior skull base (typically posterior planum sphenoidale) using a wire pass, and the galeal-pericranial graft is sutured into place with 4–0 nonresorbable sutures. The graft is often longer than the skull base defect, but the redundant tissue can be folded to make a thicker skull base reconstruction. If an open nasal approach has been used, the galeal-pericranial graft is sutured to the skull base from the nasal side to ensure a complete seal. Otherwise the endoscope can be used to ensure the galeal pericranial graft covers the dural repair if the repair is performed from the cranial side. Extended resections, such as the type 3 infratemporal fossa resection, resulting in larger skull base defects, require free-flap reconstructions with a rectus abdominis flap. Smaller defects can be closed with radial forearm flaps or even omental grafts. Regardless of whether a free flap is required, the anterior skull base defect and dural repair routinely are reconstructed with the galeal-pericranial graft over the anterior dural repair.

The craniotomy flap is replaced with a rigid plating system. A drain is placed in the epidural space through the bur hole cover and connected to a Jackson-Pratt (JP) bulb suction. This drain facilitates removal of air in the event of postoperative pneumocephalus and the potential resultant complications. The nose is packed with Xeroform gauze (Covidien, Massachusetts) to facilitate intranasal hemostasis, promote mucosal healing, and most importantly, to prevent pneumocephalus by occluding the nasal air space.

POSTOPERATIVE MANAGEMENT

Postoperative management is institution dependent, and several strategies are effective, but our current practice has evolved to minimize the postoperative complications of cerebrospinal fluid (CSF) leak and pneumocephalus. Patients are treated in the intensive care unit until the lumbar drain is removed. Lumbar drainage typically is initiated on the day after surgery at 10 mL/h and continued for 48–72 hours. The epidural drain is placed to JP bulb suction and reinflated every 30 minutes until it holds suction. The lumbar drain is typically discontinued on the morning of day 4 followed by the epidural drain 6 hours later to ensure that pneumocephalus is not induced by an unregulated leak into the lumbar drain site. The nasal packing typically is discontinued on day 5–7. Triple antibiotics are maintained until the packing is removed.

Complication Avoidance

Advances in surgical techniques and reconstruction have redefined the indications and outcomes in craniofacial reconstruction.[10] Despite this redefinition, craniofacial resection still carries significant perioperative risk and complications. Complications can be divided into several subtypes: intracranial or neurologic, extracranial or wound, and systemic or orbital. Intracranial complications include cerebrospinal fluid leak, meningitis, subdural or intradural abscess, pneumocephalus, neurologic dysfunction, subdural or extradural hematoma, cerebrovascular accident, or seizure. Extradural complications include wound infections, dehiscence, necrosis, or flap failure. Systemic complications can involve the respiratory, cardiovascular, hematologic, or endocrine systems. Orbital complications include corneal abrasion, epiphora, ectropion, enophthalmos, diplopia, periorbital cellulitis, and loss of vision. With meticulous attention to techniques of resection and reconstruction, the morbidity and mortality have been reduced; however, the complexity of skull base resection in which the intracranial space communicates with the colonized, aerated intranasal space remains a significant challenge in malignant tumors. Trouble shooting complications to minimize the impact on morbidity is essential.

INFECTION/WOUND

Infection and wound complications remain the most frequently encountered postoperative complication. In reports from the International Collaborative Study and review of the literature, Ganly and colleagues,[5] reported an overall wound complication rate of 19.6%, which was consistent with a mean overall wound complication rate of 19.8% based on a review of several previously reported complication rates.[14–17] The presence of a medical comorbidity and prior radiation were independent significant predictors of wound complications ($P<.005$).[18] Dias and colleagues[16] reported that infectious complications occurred in 38.5% of all anterior skull base cases and accounted for 54.7% of all complications. Rates of infectious complications range from 1.3% to 27.9%.[18] Osteomyelitis of the frontal bone flap occurs in 0%–14.8% of cases.[18] Earlier reports of craniofacial resection reported intracranial infection as the most frequent complication. Reviews by Boyle and colleagues[19] and Cantu and colleagues[20] of several large series found that a disproportionate amount of perioperative mortalities occurred from meningitis or intracranial abscess. However, more recent literature reports a 0%–7.7% risk of meningitis and a 0%–11% rate of intracranial abscess.[5,14,16,17,20,21] Recently, we have seen delayed brain abscesses at 1–2 years after surgery. These abscesses have been managed with stereotactic needle aspiration and prolonged antibiotics.

Several factors have contributed to a reduction in infectious complications, including shorter operating times and wrapping the bone flap in a bacitracin-soaked gauze for the duration of the surgery. The most significant factor was a change in antibiotic regimens from a single antibiotic regimen to broad-spectrum coverage with a triple antibiotic regimen using vancomycin, ceftazidime, and metronidazole, as reported by Kraus and colleagues[22] The development of a standardized perioperative antibiotic regimen has led to significant reductions in both infectious and wound-related complications. In our previously reported experience,[22] the implementation of a standardized broad-range regimen covering gram-positive, gram-negative, and anaerobic bacteria (vancomycin, ceftazidime, and metronidazole) when compared with nonstandardized regimens improved local wound complication rates from 35% to 18% and infectious wound complication rates to 11% compared with 29% in the nonstandardized arm.

In addition to changes in perioperative antibiotics, surgical techniques have also contributed to lower infectious complication rates. Neurosurgical literature recommends stripping of the frontal sinuses and packing of the frontal sinus before durotomy. Others have described the use of synthetic bone or split calvarial graft for skull base reconstruction.[23] However, the vascularized galeal-pericranial graft has been sufficient for skull base repair and helps avoid the presence of nonvascularized bone adjacent to the nasal cavity. Split calvarial graft is used to reconstruct the orbit to prevent pulsatile exophthalmos but is enveloped in vascularized galeal-pericranial graft. Over a 2-year period, we used fibrin glue as a sealant at the skull base but experienced several infections in the area of application. Our recommendation is to avoid thrombin glue, because it may act as a nidus for delayed bacterial infection.

As previously mentioned, reconstructive advances have been essential in the prevention of infectious complications, because they serve as a formidable barrier between the intracranial space and sinonasal tract. In addition to antibiotics, Kraus and colleagues[22] reported the use of a free-flap reconstruction associated with significant reduction in the rate of infectious complications: 8.2% when free flap was used compared with 27% when alternate methods of reconstruction were used.

Wound complications caused by flap failure can be prevented with meticulous surgical technique as well as careful postoperative management. Vigilant flap monitoring is conducted hourly with an external Doppler probe and in buried flaps with an internal Doppler probe. In addition, the use of vascularized free flaps as supposed to previously oft-used pedicled flaps allows for superior and appropriately sized reconstruction.

CSF LEAK

Often reported with wound complications, noninfectious cerebrospinal fluid leak remains the second most common complication, with rates reported between 3% and 20%.[24] The presentation of CSF leak typically consists of rhinorrhea and orthostatic headaches. Additionally, patients may complain of nausea, tinnitus, hearing and vision disturbances, and even facial numbness or upper extremity radicular symptoms. Rhinorrhea is typically obvious, but its presence may not be immediately evident if the nose is packed with Xeroform and the CSF is mixed with blood products. A high index of suspicion should be maintained.

Prevention of CSF leak is accomplished with meticulous watertight closure of the skull base dura. In the early descriptions of the techniques for dural closure, the dural slits created by resecting the dura from the crista galli and cribriform plate were sutured primarily. In our experience, this strategy often is unsuccessful because of the need for more extensive dural resection and the propensity to create dural rents. Dural substitutes for large defects include pericranium, alloderm, bovine pericardium, and DuraGen. Pericranium is readily available but difficult to suture because of its delicate nature and tendency to fold on itself. A bovine pericardial patch graft is ideal for dural reconstruction because it can be sutured water tight, and the edges are easily identifiable for suturing. Most importantly, in our experience, it is remarkably resistant to infection or colonization. As an added measure of prophylaxis, a DuraGen inlay graft is used as a gasket seal before suturing the bovine pericardial patch graft. This seal may help prevent a CSF leak from small suture holes or an irreparable tear of a suture line. If a CSF leak is visualized after dural reconstruction, the site should be identified, because this is almost surely a problem postoperatively, even with spinal drainage. Any site that leaks is reinforced with at temporalis muscle graft.

To help facilitate a water-tight closure, lumbar drainage of CSF is instituted at 10 mL/h by intermittently opening the stopcock and then clamping when the desired amount has drained. With continued leak, drainage is increased to 15–20 mL/h. This strategy often helps seal the leak without the need to re-explore the repair either endoscopically or via a craniotomy.

PNEUMOCEPHALUS

Pneumocephalus implies a dural defect that allows air to pass from the sinonasal into the intracranial space. When clinically significant, pneumocephalus can cause severe neurologic deficits and even result in death.

The presence of pneumocephalus implies a CSF leak in communication with an aerated space, in this case the nasal passages or sinuses. Prevention of tension pneumocephalus rests with the ability to achieve a meticulous watertight dural closure or to occlude the air space. Although it most commonly occurs from a durotomy at the skull base, it must be recognized that a CSF leak anywhere along the neuraxis can cause pneumocephalus. Lumbar drainage can promote pneumocephalus, but controlled CSF drainage at 10 mL/h rarely results in significant problems. In the setting of postoperative pneumocephalus, the lumbar drain should be clamped. Uncommonly, when the lumbar drain is discontinued, an unregulated leak of spinal fluid can occur in the low back, causing an acute decompensation from tension pneumocephalus and brain herniation. In the even that this occurs, the patient should be placed in Trendelenburg and a lumbar blood patch placed. Our current practice is to place lumbar blood patches prophylactically after discontinuation of the lumbar drain in high-risk patients.

To prevent or treat pneumocephalus, an epidural drain is placed to JP bulb suction at the time of surgery. This simple device is effective for evacuating air in the event of tension pneumocephalus.

The drain can be used to remove residual air at the end of the operation and typically will not hold suction for several hours after surgery. The JP allows for more aggressive lumbar drainage to seal a potential leak because it reduces the probability of tension pneumocephalus. On rare occasions, in our practice, the epidural drain has been used to evacuate air and reverse significant neurologic symptoms and brain herniation. Alternatively, a drain can be place through a bur hole postoperatively to evacuate air. The drain should be kept to JP bulb suction or a low suction reservoir. High-pressure reservoirs can create significant negative pressure leading to headaches, brain edema, or exacerbation of neurologic symptoms.

A third measure to prevent or treat pneumocephalus is occlusion of the air space. The nose is packed with Xeroform or Vaseline gauze (Covidien, Massachusetts). Nonocclusive packing, such as nasal tampons, is not nearly as effective. Although rarely necessary, airway control via intubation or tracheostomy can be used to reduce intracranial air extravasation. Free-flap reconstruction also facilitates occlusion of the air space but should be done in conjunction with primary dural repair. A recent patient had acute pneumocephalus with associated significant cognitive changes while flying to Europe for vacation. This event occurred 9 years after a craniofacial resection with galeal-pericranial reconstruction for esthesioneuroblastoma. No CSF leak was identified on endoscopic inspection. After repeated aspirations without successful resolution, an omental free flap was placed to occlude the nasal cavity and skull base with complete resolution of the pneumocephalus. (**Fig. 3**).

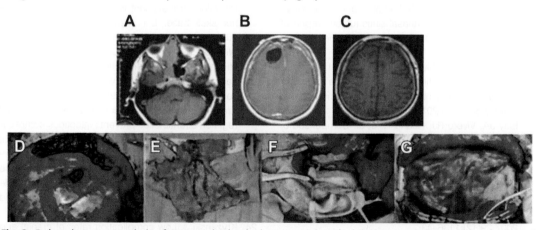

Fig. 3. Delayed pneumocephalus from resorbed galeal pericranial graft. (*A*) MR image shows right nasoethencidal esthesioneuroblastoma. (*B*) MR image shows delayed pneumocephalus. (*C*) Resolution of pneumocephalus with omental flap. (*D–G*) Intraoperative photographs of intracranial skull base repair base exposure. (*D*) Resorbed galeal pericranial graft. (*E*) Harvested omentum. (*F*) Anastomosis of superficial temporal vessels. (*G*) In-laid graft. (*Adapted from* Bilsky MH, Bentz B, Vitaz T, et al. Craniofacial resection for cranial base malignancies involving the infratemporal fossa. Neurosurgery 2005;57(4):339–47; with permission.)

SUMMARY

Combined anterior and anterolateral craniofacial resection remains the gold standard for the extirpation of skull base malignancies. Although purely endoscopic techniques are gaining traction for benign tumors, significant anatomic constraints, limitations regarding skull base repair, and the inability to achieve negative margins limit their effectiveness in the treatment of malignant tumors. The techniques of anterior and anterolateral skull base resection have evolved, as has the reconstruction using galeal-pericranial grafts combined with free-flap reconstruction when indicated. Complications are common, but meticulous attention to dural closure and early diagnosis and treatment can limit the significant morbidity associated with these procedures.

REFERENCES

1. Ketcham AS, Wilkins RH, Vanburen JM, et al. A combined intracranial facial approach to the paranasal sinuses. Am J Surg 1963;106:698–703.
2. Gil Z, Fliss DM, Cavel O, et al. Improvement in survival during the past 4 decades among patients with anterior skull base cancer. Head Neck 2012; 34(9):1212–7.
3. Patel SG, Singh B, Polluri A, et al. Craniofacial surgery for malignant skull base tumors: report of an international collaborative study. Cancer 2003; 98(6):1179–87.
4. Gil Z, Patel SG, Singh B, et al. Analysis of prognostic factors in 146 patients with anterior skull base sarcoma: an international collaborative study. Cancer 2007;110(5):1033–41.
5. Ganly I, Patel SG, Singh B, et al. Craniofacial resection for malignant paranasal sinus tumors: report of an International Collaborative Study. Head Neck 2005;27(7):575–84.
6. Raza SM, Garzon-Muvdi T, Gallia GL, et al. Craniofacial resection of midline anterior skull base malignancies: a reassessment of outcomes in the modern era. World Neurosurg 2012;78:128–36.
7. Eloy JA, Vivero RJ, Hoang K, et al. Comparison of transnasal endoscopic and open craniofacial resection for malignant tumors of the anterior skull base. Laryngoscope 2009;119(5):834–40.
8. Maghami EG, Talbot SG, Patel SG, et al. Craniofacial surgery for nonmelanoma skin malignancy: report of an international collaborative study. Head Neck 2007;29(12):1136–43.
9. Soler ZM, Smith TL. Endoscopic versus open craniofacial resection of esthesioneuroblastoma: what is the evidence? Laryngoscope 2012;122(2): 244–5.
10. Bilsky MH, Bentz B, Vitaz T, et al. Craniofacial resection for cranial base malignancies involving the infratemporal fossa. Neurosurgery 2005;57(Suppl 4): 339–47 [discussion: 339–47].
11. Sen C, Triana A, Hiltzik D, et al. Malignant tumors involving the lateral skull base. Clin Neurosurg 2001;48:373–86.
12. Bigelow DC, Smith PG, Leonetti JP, et al. Treatment of malignant neoplasms of the lateral cranial base with the combined frontotemporal-anterolateral approach: five-year follow-up. Otolaryngol Head Neck Surg 1999;120(1):17–24.
13. Mickey B, Close L, Schaefer S, et al. A combined frontotemporal and lateral infratemporal fossa approach to the skull base. J Neurosurg 1988;68(5):678–83.
14. Ketcham AS, Van Buren JM. Tumors of the paranasal sinuses: a therapeutic challenge. Am J Surg 1985;150(4):406–13.
15. Janecka IP, Sen C, Sekhar LN, et al. Cranial base surgery: results in 183 patients. Otolaryngol Head Neck Surg 1994;110(6):539–46.
16. Dias FL, Sa GM, Kligerman J, et al. Complications of anterior craniofacial resection. Head Neck 1999; 21(1):12–20.
17. Donald PJ. Complications in skull base surgery for malignancy. Laryngoscope 1999;109(12):1959–66.
18. Ganly I, Patel SG, Singh B, et al. Complications of craniofacial resection for malignant tumors of the skull base: report of an International Collaborative Study. Head Neck 2005;27(6):445–51.
19. Boyle JO, Shah KC, Shah JP. Craniofacial resection for malignant neoplasms of the skull base: an overview. J Surg Oncol 1998;69(4):275–84.
20. Cantu G, Riccio S, Bimbi G, et al. Craniofacial resection for malignant tumours involving the anterior skull base. Eur Arch Otorhinolaryngol 2006; 263(7):647–52.
21. Wellman BJ, Traynelis VC, McCulloch TM, et al. Midline anterior craniofacial approach for malignancy: results of en bloc versus piecemeal resections. Skull Base Surg 1999;9(1):41–6.
22. Kraus DH, Gonen M, Mener D, et al. A standardized regimen of antibiotics prevents infectious complications in skull base surgery. Laryngoscope 2005; 115(8):1347–57.
23. Raza SM, Quinones-Hinojosa A, Lim M, et al. The transconjunctival transorbital approach: a keyhole approach to the midline anterior skull base. World Neurosurg 2012.
24. Kryzanski J. Low complication rates of cranial and craniofacial approaches to midline anterior skull base lesions. Skull Base 2008;18(4):229–41.

Minimally Invasive Approaches to the Anterior Skull Base

Michael E. Ivan, MD[a,b], Arman Jahangiri, BS[a,b],
Ivan H. El-Sayed, MD[b,c], Manish K. Aghi, MD, PhD[a,b,*]

KEYWORDS

- Minimally invasive surgery • Endoscopy • Skull base malignancy • Anterior craniofacial

KEY POINTS

- The advantages of minimally invasive endoscopic approaches to the skull base are: (1) devascularization of the skull base blood supply before tumor resection, (2) avoidance of brain manipulation and retraction, (3) protecting the vascular supply of the optic apparatus as the tumor is approached from below by maintaining arachnoid planes, and (4) providing a better cosmetic result.
- Limitations of minimally invasive approaches include: (1) instrumentation that may be associated with greater application of force on surrounding structures than when using microinstruments; (2) difficulty accessing large tumors with significant lateral extension; (3) difficulty resecting the entire dural attachment, potentially limiting gross total resections; (4) difficulty with resection of tumor that completely encase vascular structures; and (5) lack of three-dimensional visualization.
- Selection of the appropriate minimally invasive approach depends on identification of the appropriate entry point and surgical corridor.
- Through careful surgical planning to avoid complications and select appropriate patients, minimally invasive techniques can be used to improve the function and prognosis of patients with skull base malignancies.

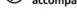 Videos of "Exposure of and removal of anterior skull base dura" and "Anterior skull base closure" accompany this article. at http://www.neurosurgery.theclinics.com/

INTRODUCTION

Minimally invasive approaches in neurosurgery have been a recent, yet rapidly growing area that is becoming a more accepted and valuable tool in the neurosurgeon's armamentarium. This area continues to rapidly expand because of continual developments in technique and equipment, most specifically endoscopy. As with any new field, these minimally invasive approaches are not always intuitive and require additional training and time to develop the needed skills. Once acquired, however, minimally invasive approaches have been shown to decrease morbidity and speed recovery in patients while providing similar extent of resection.

This article reviews the tenets of the minimally invasive approaches to the anterior skull base in neurosurgery and discusses the history of this technique, advantages and disadvantages, the corridors and pathways of the approaches, the equipment and operating room setup, perioperative care, and complication avoidance.

HISTORY

Skull base surgery has been founded on the ideals of finding the most direct access to skull based

Disclosure: A.J. is a Howard Hughes Medical Institute (HHMI) Research Fellow.
[a] Department of Neurological Surgery, University of California San Francisco, 505 Parnassus Avenue, CA 94143-0112, USA; [b] Center for Minimally Invasive Skull Base Surgery, University of California San Francisco, 505 Parnassus Avenue, CA 94143-0112, USA; [c] Department of Otolaryngology–Head and Neck Surgery, University of California San Francisco, 505 Parnassus Avenue, CA 94143-0112, USA
* Corresponding author. 505 Parnassus Avenue, M-774, Box 0112, San Francisco, CA 94143-0112.
E-mail address: aghim@neurosurg.ucsf.edu

Neurosurg Clin N Am 24 (2013) 19–37
http://dx.doi.org/10.1016/j.nec.2012.08.001
1042-3680/13/$ – see front matter © 2013 Elsevier Inc. All rights reserved.

lesions with the least amount of risk and brain manipulation. The first attempts at anterior skull based surgery were likely performed by the ancient Egyptians as evidence by intranasal dissection found in their remains.[1] However, not until 1894 was the transphenoidal approach first discussed when David Giordano performed an anatomical study via a transfacial transphenoidal exposure to gain access to the sella turcia.[2] Then in 1907, the first transphenoidal resection of a pituitary tumor was performed by Hermann Schloffer in Austria.[3] Theodor Kocher and Oskar Hirsh further modified the procedure by developing submucosal removal of the septum and an endonasal transseptal transphenoidal procedure that then set the stage for Harvey Cushing to later improve.[3–5] Harvey Cushing, who completed more than 231 pituitary surgeries via a sublabial transphenoidal approach, had an astonishingly low mortality rate of 5.6% during his career.[5] At the same time, the mortality rates of larger open transfrontal surgeries to access the anterior skull base were also decreasing and ultimately equaled that of the more difficult transphenoidal approach. Therefore popularity for these challenging minimally invasive approaches declined until the inventions of the intraoperative radiofluoroscopy and the operating microscope in the 1950's-1960's.[3,6] Jules Hardy, who was responsible for the first use of the operating microscope during the transphenoidal approach, spread the teaching of this approach throughout North America. He was responsible for the development of many of the micro-instruments used in transphenoidal surgery.[3] With continued advancements in technology and technique, the methods that Hardy developed continue to improve and have resulted in minimally invasive procedures of the anterior skull base becoming accepted as an effective and safe procedure.

The first neurosurgical endoscopic surgery was performed in 1910 by Lespinasse. Lespinasse, who practiced urology, performed choroid plexus coagulation via a burr hole in two children with hydrocephalus. In 1923, the neurosurgeons, William Mixter and Walter Dandy, performed the first endoscopic third ventriculoscopy; however, this procedure was severely limited by poor visualization.[7,8] The use of endoscopy in neurosurgery was not well accepted until improvements were made in the endoscopes and additional supportive equipment, as well as in the understanding of the surrounding microanatomy. The return of endoscopy in neurosurgery did not occur until the late twentieth century. Gerard Guiot, in 1963, was likely the first neurosurgeon to apply the endoscope to transsphenoidal surgery. He soon abandoned its use, however, due to poor visualization and light compared with the operative microscope.[8,9] Then in the 1990s, endoscopy increased independently with otorhinolaryngologists operating on the paranasal sinuses for the treatment of inflammatory sinonasal disorders.[10] Then, with the collaboration of these two disciplines, there began a new era in surgical technique with the use of the endoscopy. With the addition of angled lens, surgeons were now able to see areas that were previously unreachable with such small exposure. In 1992, Jankowski and colleagues[11] and, in 1995, Sethi and Pillay[12] (otorhinolaryngologists and neurosurgeons) reported the use of the endonasal endoscopy transsphenoidal technique that relied solely on the use of the endoscope for complete visualization during surgery. With improved lighting, optics, and high-definition imaging, expanded endoscopic techniques have become routine in the management of complex sinonasal and anterior skull base surgery and have also spread to spinal surgery, peripheral nerve surgery, craniosynostosis correction, aneurysm clipping, and accessing of ventricular masses.

Management of anterior skull base lesions endoscopically advanced significantly with the advent of two-surgeon expanded endonasal approaches.[13] In this set up, two surgeons work in tandem to using a four-handed technique to maintain surgical visualization while dissecting with two instruments. At the skull base, an otorhinolaryngologist and neurosurgeon work to dissect tumor from the dura and anterior cranial fossa. Adequate closure of the skull-base defects with the pedicle axial vascularized nasoseptal flap (NSF) has reduced the cerebral spinal fluid (CSF)-leak rate and allowed rapid expansion of endonasal techniques.[14] With advances in minimally invasive techniques continuing to develop, surgeons can customize an approach for each patient and their disease to allow for the safest and most effective treatment.

Keyhole Surgery

The supraorbital craniotomy offers a window to the inferior frontal lobe, to the circle of Willis, and dissection of the sylvian fissure without the need of brain retraction.[15,16] In 1912, McArthur[17] reported trephination following incision over the eyebrow. In 1913, Frazier[18] described the supraorbital approach to treat a pituitary adenoma in the anterior fossa. In 1984, Jane and colleagues[19] used the supraorbital approach to treat orbital tumors, anterior communicating artery aneurysms, pituitary adenomas, craniopharyngiomas, and parasellar or olfactory groove meningiomas. With the advent of neuronavigation and improved microsurgical instrumentation in the 1990s, the supraorbital keyhole approach has become a more accepted approach to anterior communicating artery aneurysms, pituitary tumors, and craniopharyngiomas.[20,21]

ADVANTAGES OF MINIMALLY INVASIVE APPROACHES

Traditional open approaches to the anterior skull base include bifrontal craniotomies, extended bifrontal craniotomies, pterional craniotomies, as well as complex transfacial operations. These approaches, while adequate, require a large incision, and significant brain exposure and retraction that places critical structures at risk and increases recovery time. This exposure can also cause cosmetic defects in the forehead resulting from the incisional scar, depression of the bone flap, inadequate repair of burr holes, and/or temporal muscle atrophy.[15] With the recent application of concepts from endonasal sinus surgery, neurosurgeons, working with otolaryngologists, can obtain access with a direct anatomic route to the lesion with a minimal opening that limits brain exposure and minimizes iatrogenic trauma. Similar to the larger transcranial approach, minimally invasive approaches obviate brain retraction. Little data are published comparing complications of open verses endoscopic approaches, but the advantages seem intuitive. Proponents argue that, in contrast to the various transcranial approaches, the minimally invasive approaches: (1) devascularize the skull base blood supply before tumor resection,[22] (2) avoid brain manipulation and retraction,[23] (3) allow the intervening arachnoid plane to protect the vascular supply of the optic apparatus because the tumor is approached from below,[24] and (4) provide a better cosmetic result.[25] Typically, these minimally invasive approaches forego skin incisions; instead, the natural apertures in the face are used to gain access. Most tumors in the sinonasal cavity that involve the anterior skull base, and many lesions emanating directly from the anterior skull base, grow in a mediolateral direction, displacing structures laterally, which creates natural corridors that allows resection via an anteromedial approach.

DISADVANTAGES OF MINIMALLY INVASIVE APPROACHES

Minimally invasive approaches are often deemed difficult because they require increased knowledge of anatomy, particularly anatomy outside the cranial compartment; experience with a different set of instruments that often must be handled further from the site of the pathologic condition; and decreased working room for the surgeon.[26] Although many improvements in techniques and

instruments have occurred over the past decades, surgeons must have knowledge about the limitations in using minimally invasive techniques. Attention must be paid to (1) instrumentation that may be associated with greater application of force on surrounding structures than when using microinstruments, (2) difficulty accessing large tumors with significant lateral extension,[24] (3) difficulty resecting of the entire dural attachment, potentially limiting gross total resections (GTRs),[24] (4) resection of tumor that completely encase vascular structures, and (5) lack of three-dimensional visualization.[24] Another drawback of a minimally invasive approach is the inability to quickly adapt to unexpected findings or intraoperative catastrophes through a limited opening. Therefore, complete preoperative imaging, careful patient selection, and thorough surgical planning are of the utmost importance.[15] In addition, high leaks of CSF have been reported with minimally invasive approaches, which, if they persistent, can lead to other complications. It has been suggested that a surgeon should not choose a minimally invasive approach if a tumor typically extends greater than 1 cm beyond the exposure, which could restrict obtaining a GTR.[27] However, surgical classification is currently a moving target as techniques and surgical experience increase. In some cases, intracranial pressure will help express the tumor downwards toward the skull base as the inferior bulk of tumor is resected. This allows for resection of tumors that have extended further intracranially. In these cases, having the option of an open approach or a combined approach may allow a more extensive resection and provide a better patient care. Anatomic constraints, such as encasement of significant vessels or extension beyond the plane of cranial nerve or major vessel, limit endoscopic selection. In general, consent for a possible open approach should be discussed with the patient preoperatively. In particular, lateral spread along the dura should be evaluated on MRI preoperatively. Additional cautions to consider include extent of tumor invasion into the brain, tumor vascularity, patient age and comorbidities, surgeon expertise, and resources.[28]

EXAMPLES OF MALIGNANT OR POTENTIALLY MALIGNANT ANTERIOR SKULL BASE TUMOR ACCESSIBLE THROUGH A MINIMALLY INVASIVE APPROACH

Most of the malignant lesions located in the anterior skull base consists of rare tumors that present in an aggressive invasive stage. Therefore, much of the literature on skull base malignancies is characterized by single-institution experiences with a variety of tumor locations, histology, and treatment planes, with the rarity of the pathologies making it difficult to draw firm conclusions about prognosis or the role for minimally invasive approaches in the resection.

The most common lesions in the anterior skull base include pituitary adenomas, spontaneous CSF leaks, meningiomas, and craniopharyngiomas.[27] These lesions are benign, yet often require surgical intervention in which minimally invasive approaches are typically used. Less common lesions in the anterior skull base include chordoma, Rathke cleft cysts, and esthesioneuroblastoma. Finally, the very rare lesions found in the skull base include, but are not limited to, pituitary carcinoma, metastasis, hemangiopericytoma, rhabdomyosarcoma, adenoid cystic carcinoma, malignant salivary gland tumor, juvenile angiofibroma, schwannoma, enterogenous cyst, osteoma, papilloma, nasal glioma, lipoma, gout, and rheumatoid pannus.[27] Although meningiomas and craniopharyngiomas are classified as benign tumors, they can be aggressive (particularly craniopharyngioma) due to their invasion and propensity to recur if not fully treated. Meningioma is the most common anterior skull base tumor and can be located at three specific locations of the anterior skull base from anterior to posterior: olfactory groove, planum sphenoidale, and tuberculum sellae. A surgeon must ensure that with minimally invasive techniques they can still achieve the lowest possible Simpson grade.[29] Tumors that have large dural tails, or extend laterally, may be better treated with larger, open approaches. Treatment options include monitoring of small, slow-growing lesions, radiation, or surgical resection. The most common surgical complication is cranial nerve palsies.[30] Craniopharyngiomas, which originate from pituitary embryonic tissue and are lined with squamous epithelium, are typically found in the sellar or suprasellar regions. These tumors occur mostly in children and are less frequent in the adult population. Preoperative and postoperative endocrinologic evaluation is necessary to assess for hypopituitarism, as well as a full evaluation of visual fields. Treatment includes surgical resection and, if residual tumor is noted, potential adjuvant radiation.[31]

Malignant tumors of the anterior skull base can be divided into neuroendocrine sinonasal malignancies and non-neuroendocrine sino-nasopharyngeal tumors. Neuroendocrine sinonasal malignancies originate from epithelium of the paranasal sinuses and can spread to the anterior cranial fossa. These include esthesioneuroblastomas and nonesthesioneuroblastomas (ie, neuroendocrine carcinomas, sinonasal undifferentiated carcinoma [SNUC], and small cell carcinomas).

Non-neuroendocrine sino-nasopharyngeal tumors also spread to the anterior cranial fossa and include adenoid cystic carcinomas, squamous cell carcinoma, adenocarcinoma, sarcoma, and melanoma.

Neuroendocrine Group of Sinonasal Malignancies

Esthesioneuroblastomas
Esthesioneuroblastomas, or olfactory neuroblastomas, arise from the olfactory epithelium of the upper nasal cavity and compromise 3% of intracranial tumors. They have a binomial distribution, affect patients in their second and fifth decade of life, and are thought to be a primal neuroectodermal tumor.[32] Esthesioneuroblastomas often invades into the cranial vault and, to assist with prognostic factors, radiographically the tumor is divided into Kadish stages.[33] This radiographic grading scale is as follows[33]:

A—limited to nasal cavity.

B—nasal and paranasal cavity.

C—beyond nasal and paranasal cavity (invades cribriform plate, anterior cranial base or orbit, intracranial, and maxillary sinus).

In a meta-analysis comparing surgery as a unimodal treatment versus surgery plus irradiation there was no significant difference. In patients who underwent surgery alone, instead of surgery plus irradiation, the survival rate at 5 years was 78% versus 75% and, at 10 years, was 67% versus 61%.[34] Further analysis showed that poor prognostic indicators were a Kadish grade of C, more invasive tumor type, and patients greater than 65 years of age.[34] Resection of these tumors is extensive and the goal is negative margins, which can include excision of the cribriform plate and overlying dura (**Figs. 1** and **2**, Video 1). Typically, biopsying the tumor before complete excision is recommended to establish the diagnosis and determine whether there is a role for pre-resection chemotherapy and/or radiation treatment to achieve cytoreduction before definitive resection.[34] Other studies show variable results with 5-year survival rates ranging from 56% to 100%.[35–37]

Non-esthesioneuroblastoma neuroendocrine malignancies
SNUC SNUC is an aggressive tumor that originates in the paranasal sinuses. This malignancy is usually present in an aggressive stage with local and distant metastases. No current consensus on the optimal treatment exists owing to the rarity of this disease and poor outcomes; however, a combination of resection, chemotherapy, and radiotherapy has been shown to improve survival rates.[38,39] The University of California San Francisco experience

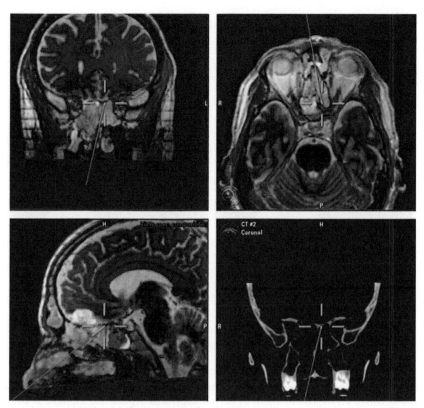

Fig. 1. Intraoperative neuronavigation for resection of esthesioneuroblastoma. Preoperative MRI and CT scan fused for intraoperative navigation in a patient diagnosed with an esthesioneuroblastoma. This lesion was resected endoscopically and the patient has been disease-free for 3 years.

with 19 patients incorporating radiation therapy and surgery revealed a 74%, 5-year, local control rate if a GTR was achieved compared with only a 24% local control rate for those with subtotal tumor resection.[40]

A recent meta-analysis revealed that survival of patients with SNUC at 23 months was approximately 47%.[39] Recent data in a small series suggest that minimally invasive endoscopic gross-total resection of an SNUC with adjuvant therapy in patients without metastases can allow a disease-free survival rate of 57% at 32 months from diagnosis.[38]

Sinonasal neuroendocrine carcinoma Like SNUC, sinonasal neuroendocrine carcinoma (SNEC) is an aggressive tumor, usually presenting in middle age as a nasal mass. Both tumors have the capacity to metastasize locally and distantly, and typically result in poor outcomes. SNEC, which is even rarer than SNUC, has been described in small, single-institution series.[41]

Small cell carcinoma Small cell carcinoma typically present aggressively. It is even rarer than SNUC and SNEC, and has been described in small series.[42]

Non-Neuroendocrine Sino-Nasopharyngeal Tumors

Nasopharyngeal carcinomas

Adenoid cystic carcinoma of the salivary glands Adenoid cystic carcinoma is also a rare cancer that can occur at multiple sites in the body but most often occurs in the head and neck. At this location this tumor is considered to be a malignant salivary gland tumor. Adenoid cystic carcinoma starts in the maxillary sinus and invades neural foramen. Typically, complete resection is not possible owing to perineural extension, especially into cranial nerves V2 and V3.[32] The goal of surgery is to resect as much as possible without compromising the orbit or cranial nerves. The primary treatment is surgical resection followed by postoperative radiation treatment.[32] Chemotherapy is also used for metastatic disease. In one study of 160 patients, 5-year survival rates were 89% to 90% and 15-year survival rates were 40% to 69%.[43,44] In 22% of the patients, the site of failure was a distant metastasis.[43] Increased mortality and treatment failures were associated with positive lymph nodes, solid histology, and perineural invasion.[43]

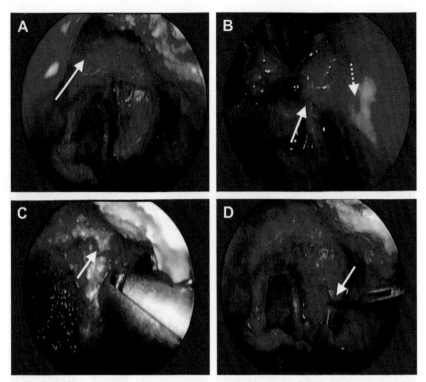

Fig. 2. Resection of esthesioneuroblastoma. (*A*) Exposure of posterior wall of frontal sinuses delineates anterior extent of resection (*white arrow*). (*B*) Removal of lamina papyracea exposes the ethmoid artery entering skull base (*white solid arrow*), the periorbita is retracted (*dotted arrow*). (*C*) After drilling down the skull base, the bone (*arrow*) is further resected with a Kerrison rongeur. (*D*) Dural margins are defined and resected with retraction and endoscopic scissors (*arrow*).

Squamous cell carcinoma Squamous cell carcinomas are the most common malignancies of the nose and paranasal sinuses and tend to present in men over the age of 50. Treatment plans include surgery, radiation treatment, or both, depending on the grade of the stage of the tumor.[32] In a meta-analysis reviewing 89 patients who underwent resection for squamous cell carcinomas, the 2-year disease-free rate was 64%.[45]

Primary sinus (adenocarcinoma, sarcoma) or sinonasal (melanoma) pathology
Sinonasal melanoma Sinonasal melanoma or mucosa melanoma is very rare, accounting for only 1% of all melanomas. Tumors often present in late-stage disease with extension from the sinuses into the skull base. Treatment consists of aggressive surgical resection and subsequent adjuvant radiotherapy.[46] In a study of 53 patients, the 3-year survival was reported as 28% and the recurrence-free survival was 25%.[46]

Sinus sarcoma Sarcomas in the head and neck are also very rare and present as a late diagnosis, making their prognosis poor. Low-grade tumors are treated primarily with irradiation, whereas high grade is treated with combination surgery and irradiation, as well as chemotherapy.[32]

Other Anterior Skull Base Aggressive Lesions
Other malignant anterior skull base lesions can include rare more aggressive forms of usually benign intracranial lesions such as atypical or malignant meningioma, or pituitary carcinoma. Finally, there are tumors that are pathologically benign, which can ultimately prove fatal owing to frequent recurrence (eg, suprasellar craniopharyngiomas or infrasellar chordomas). Chordomas are persistent fetal cartilage and notochords involved in skull base development that give rise to their malignant counterparts, chondrosarcomas and chordomas, respectively. Their incidence is 0.8 per 100,000 and they comprise approximately 0.1% of all brain tumors. Chordomas are histologically benign and slow-growing; however, they are considered malignant because of their tendency to engulf and invade neurovascular structures. The origins of these two tumors lead to different locations, with chordomas arising in midline

notochord-derived locations (eg, clivus), whereas chondrosarcomas arise from cartilaginous lateral skull base. Their midline location makes chordomas an appealing target for an endonasal endoscopic approach. During resection of these lesions, neuromonitoring is critical, especially due to the medial course cranial nerve VI takes around the clivus. Treatment of these lesions begins with surgical resection, followed with early adjuvant irradiation (either gamma knife or proton beam). In a review of 12 endonasal series, GTR was achieved in 40% to 72%.[47–56] Limitations preventing GTR included tumor volume greater than 20 cm^3, tumor location in lower clivus with lateral extension, and previously treated disease.[50] In one study of 60 resected endonasal, endoscopic chordomas, 20% of patients who underwent GTR had recurrence at 15.4 months and 60% of patients who underwent subtotal resection had recurrence at 13.7 months.[50]

ANTERIOR SKULL BASE CORRIDORS, APPROACHES, AND TARGETS

Minimally invasive anterior skull base approaches have been continually developed by neurosurgeons and otolaryngologists working together over many years and can allow access from the olfactory groove to the odontoid process of C2. The best way to preserve collateral structures is to not expose them. Wide exposure of the brain and vascular structures to the surgical field to nonphysiological conditions for several hours is undesirable. Therefore, the purpose of a minimally invasive approach is to pinpoint where the lesion is and choose a short, direct, targeted approach that eliminates such wide exposures used in the traditional approaches. To find such a selected approach, the surgeon must be familiar and comfortable with three-dimensional skull base anatomy. In addition, the preoperative imaging must be vigilantly reviewed to see where structures are compressed and altered from their original location.

When planning the surgical approach, the surgeon decides on the target, the corridor, and an entry point.[27] The approach should minimize the need for manipulating any vascular or neural components.[28] At the beginning of the case, the surgeon must already be aware of the closure method that will be needed at the end of the operation. This will dictate the best way to open the mucosal layer to ensure vascular supply is preserved if a nasoseptal flap will be needed.

The decision begins with determining a target. Targets in the anterior skull base include, but are not limited to, the sinonasal cavity, the olfactory

groove, the anterior cranial fossa, the sella, the suprasellar cistern, the clivus, the cavernous sinus, the orbital apex, and the inferior frontal lobe.

The tumors at each of these targets typically start in the midline, but can grow more laterally. Understanding how much lateral projection, where the vascular supply is, and where the dural attachment is located are important in planning the next step of selecting an entry point to the skull base to best access this target. Entry points include transfrontal, transcribriform, transclival, transsellar, transtuberculum, and transplanum (**Figs. 3** and **4**). In addition, some lesions of the suprasellar areas or the inferior frontal lobe are best accessed via a supraorbital or supraglabellar approach. After an entry point is selected, a corridor through which the entry point to the skull base will be achieved is chosen. Most of the corridors to the anterior skull base begin transnasally and then extend to either include transsphenoidal and/or transethmoidal corridors (**Fig. 5**). Other corridors that are used less frequently are sublabial and transoral. These assist with gaining access to lesions that are lower in the skull base. Finally, if the lesion extends more laterally and enters the middle fossa, extension of the entry might include transmaxillary and transpterygoid approaches.

Corridors

Transnasal

Almost all entry points to the anterior skull base begin transnasally because this entry provides largest access to the skull base and is often required for the other corridors. This approach is the least invasive due to minimal soft tissue and bony disruption. The borders include the cribriform

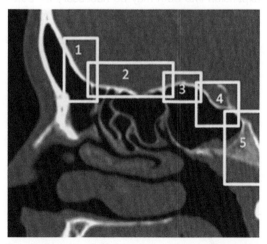

Fig. 3. Anterior skull base entry Points. Shown are examples of five anterior skull base entry points: (1) transfrontal, (2) transcribriform, (3) transtuberculum or transplanum, (4) transsellar, and (5) transclival.

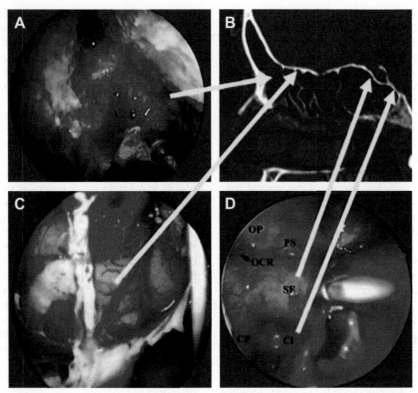

Fig. 4. Skull base views. (*A*) Frontal sinus throughout transfrontal entry point. (*B*) Location of views on the skull base (*yellow arrows*). (*C*) Olfactory nerves seen through the transcribriform entry point. (*D*) Planum sphenoidale (PS), sellar fossa (SF), and clivus (CI) as intersinus septum is being removed via the transsellar entry point. CP, carotid protuberance; OCR, optic-carotid recess; OP, optic- protuberance.

plate superiorly; the septum medially; the superior, medial, and inferior turbinates laterally; and the hard palate inferiorly.[27] Typically, for smaller cases, using one nasal passage is sufficient; however, expansion into both may be necessary for better exposure or to allow more ease of instrument manipulation.

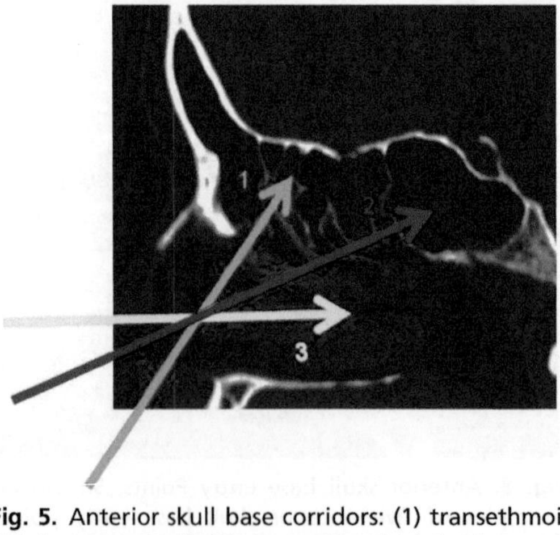

With this expansion, the surgeon removes the posterior aspects of the septum. Care must be given to not remove the septum too anteriorly because deformation of the nasal ridge can result. Additionally, removal of the middle turbinate can also decompress the intranasal compartment and allow better working space if needed. Continuing the transnasal opening posteriorly, the surgeon can access the olfactory groove, cribriform plate, and anterior cranial fossa.[27]

Transethmoidal

Once entered via the transnasal corridor, the surgeon can decide the extent of superior lateral access that is required. If needed, extension into transethmoidal area can be performed by advancing lateral to the vertical attachment of the medial turbinate. This allows complete removal of the anterior and posterior ethmoids. Exposure is then gained to the fovea ethmoidalis, frontal fossa, lamina papyracea, and orbital apex.[27] Further extension through a transsellar approach will also allow access to the cavernous sinus.

Fig. 5. Anterior skull base corridors: (1) transethmoidal (*green arrow*), (2) transsphenoidal (*red arrow*), and (3) transnasal (*yellow arrow*).

Transsphenoidal

The transsphenoidal corridor is the mainstay for basic cases and is the workhorse for pituitary lesions. After using the transnasal corridor, a large opening into the sphenoid sinus is made. One method is to enlarge the sphenoid ostia bilaterally.[27] As described above, the posterior septum is removed. The mucosal lining of the sinus are stripped, and the septations are removed. At this point, a large opening into the sphenoid sinus is achieved. Access to the sella, tuberculum sellae, planum sphenoidale, cavernous sinus, and upper third of the clivus is achieved.

Expanded Endonasal Surgical Technique

The procedure can be tailored to the lesion at hand but, in general, starts with creation of a surgical corridor to allow passage of the endoscope and at least two surgical instruments. The procedure is often initiated by the otolaryngology team. The nasal cavity is decongested preoperatively with intranasal packing of 1:1000 epinephrine or 4 mL of 4% cocaine on pledgets. Obstructing sinonasal tumors are often debrided through various means such as blunt or sharp dissection or electrocautery, which can lead to bleeding. The tumor is packed off with hemostatic agent and pledgets soaked with decongestant. A wide maxillary antrostomy and total ethmoidectomy is typically performed on the right side (unless a unilateral left dissection is being performed). Next, if planned for use, a nasal septal flap is harvested and stored in the maxillary antrum or nasopharynx. The posterior 1.5 cm is removed to provide access to lesions of the sphenoid planum and pituitary. For lesions involving the anterior cranial fossa, the entire septum may need to be removed preserving the anterior nasal L strut (approximately 1.5 cm of the anterior nasal septum) to prevent a saddle nose deformity. Variations of nasal septectomy can be tailored on a case-by-case basis, but should not obstruct surgical access. A wide sphenoidotomy is performed from orbital lamina to orbital lamina to correctly identify the plane of the orbit. Anteriorly, the frontal sinus is identified by complete removal of the anterior ethmoid cells. The authors prefer to enter the frontal sinuses in the midline using a high-speed coarse diamond burr, drilling out the nasal septum where it enters the floor of the frontal sinus. The remainder of the frontal sinus floor is removed with 70 angled Kerrison rongeur. The anterior ethmoid artery is identified traversing from the orbit to midline at the junction of the anterior skull base with the posterior wall of the frontal sinus. The posterior ethmoid artery traverses the skull base just anterior to the anterior sphenoid

sinus wall. Importantly, the ethmoids often travel within the bone of the skull base, and we prefer to identify them in the orbit. The orbit lamina bone can then be removed, preserving the periorbita to prevent herniation of orbital fat into the surgical field. The vessels are identified and ligated. The skull base bone, if intact, can then be eggshelled with a high speed burr. The crista galli is identified dividing the left and right anterior skull base, and can be drilled out from nasal cavity using a diamond burr. After the tumor is devascularized and debulked to the dura, the neurosurgical team typically joins for a meticulous tandem dissection of the intracranial disease. Typically, a clean dural margin can be identified by its pearly white appearance and using extended microdissection or microscissors, the dura is entered in a disease-free zone. The dura is dissected off the brain circumferentially around the disease. At this point, it is often appreciated that intracranial tumor can descend into the nasal cavity, facilitating dissection. If dictated for control of malignant disease, the tumor is dissected off the brain with a clean margin. After the tumor is resected, we typically close the wound with a fitted piece of DuraGen (Integra Life Sciences, Plainsboro, NJ, USA) soaked in saline, then cover the wound with the septal flap. In some cases, a fat graft can be used to supplement the closure. In some cases, if the flap is too small for the defect, we place the fat graft on the DuraGen, then vascularize the fat with the septal flap. In other cases, we have supplemented the edges of the septal flap with a fat bolster. The nasal septum is covered with Silastic splints if there is exposed cartilage. The cavity is then packed with 10 cm Merocel sponges (Medtronic Xomed, Jacksonville, FL, USA) and a Foley balloon catheter filled with saline under direct observation.

Entry Points

Transcribriform or transfrontal

The transcribriform entry point is accessed through the transnasal corridor by projecting medially and superiorly. This access allows visualization from the olfactory groove and crista galli, along the floor of the anterior fossa to the anterior planum sphenoidale.[28] More superiorly, the frontal sinus can be entered if tumor extension is present and this entry point would be transfrontal.[28] Because of the high angle of entry, a 30° endoscopic is very useful for examining beyond the floor of the anterior fossa. Typical tumor types at this location include esthesioneuroblastoma, SNUC, adenoid cystic carcinoma, olfactory groove meningiomas, and squamous cell carcinoma. If the tumor extends more laterally off midline, this approach can be expanded to include transfovea ethmoidalis approach; however, careful attention and possible transaction of the ethmoidal arteries is needed.[27] In addition, the supraorbital approach or supraglabellar approach may be better suited for tumors depending on the amount of bony involvement and location. Damage to the olfactory structures as they enter the cribriform plate bilaterally will result in anosmia; therefore, this risk should be addressed with the patient preoperatively.

Transsellar

The transsellar entry point is accessed via the transsphenoidal corridor and allows exposure to the sellar and suprasellar structures. Laterally the exposure is limited by the cavernous segment of the internal carotid artery. Most of the lesions (Rathke cleft cyst and pituitary gland) originating in sella are benign; however, the approach is needed to address inferior extension of suprasellar pathologic tumor (craniopharyngiomas) or superior extension of infrasellar pathologic tumor (chordomas). The pituitary gland can be transposed, if needed, to gain further access to superior intradural aspect of a superiorly growing chordoma. Care must be given to the location of the hypophyseal arteries; the superior artery must be preserved and, if needed, the inferior artery can be sacrificed. In addition, evaluation and removal of tumor that invades into the medial cavernous sinus can be approached with this method.[27] Finally, tumor that extends superiorly and laterally may need removal of the opticocarotid recess. This can be removed by carefully drilling until the bone is eggshell thin and then slowly elevating the bone with a rongeur such as a Cloward. Removal of tumor from surrounding the optic nerve not only allows decompression of the nerve but also a safer target for radiosurgery in the postoperative treatment.

Transtuberculum or transplanum

The transtuberculum and transplanum approaches typically involve an extension of the transsellar entry point anteriorly or the transcribriform entry point posteriorly. With this additional exposure, better visualization of the suprasellar cistern is achieved, especially when tumors are more anteriorly and superiorly projecting. The planum sphenoidale or the tuberculum are thinned out to eggshell thinness, then removed carefully with an up-biting Hardy punch. Typically, the anterior and superior wall of the sella is also removed. Through a midline dural opening, access to the optic nerves, anterior communicating artery, interhemispheric cistern, and distally third ventricle can be achieved.[27] Special attention to the superior intercavernous sinus must be made, and ligation

can be performed if it cannot be displaced. Representative pathologic conditions in this location are meningiomas, craniopharyngiomas, or large pituitary lesions with significant superior extension.[28]

Transclival

The transclival entry point is accessed via the transnasal and/or transsphenoidal corridor and allows visualization of the clivus. The clivus can then be accessed from the level of the posterior clinoids to the foramen magnum.[28] When entering the sphenoid sinus, removal of the inferior aspect of the anterior wall down to the floor of the sphenoid sinus, close to the nasopharynx, is needed to allow a more downward trajectory. Identification of the petrosal segment of the internal carotid artery in the posterior wall of the sphenoid sinus is imperative and will limit the lateral extension of resection. This bone can be drilled carefully to expose the surrounding venous plexus and carotid artery. Micro-Doppler can be used if the carotid is encased with tumor for localization. Because the clivus also extends superiorly and posteriorly to the pituitary gland, a transsellar entry point may also be needed for mobilization of the pituitary gland.[27] The tumor will likely erode a large part of the clivus, but the remaining portion can be drilled down to allow full exposure of the tumor. Again, to allow a wider corridor, resection of one or both of the middle turbinates may be needed on entry to allow access to all involved structures. If the tumor erodes into the dura, opening the dura at the midline at or below the vertebral basilar junction will allow careful preservation of cranial nerve VI as it runs laterally into Dorello canal.[49] The lateral limitation of this exposure include the vidian nerve running along the lateral border of the inferior aspect of sphenoid sinus; the carotid arteries; and, inferiorly, the eustachian tubes in the lateral nasopharynx mucosa.[27] Typical pathologic tumors at this location include chordoma, chondrosarcomas, and lymphoma.

Supraorbital Approach

The supraorbital and supraglabellar approaches offer a window to the inferior frontal lobe and the circle of Willis, and dissection of the sylvian fissure without the need of brain retraction.[15,16,57] This approach does not disturb the temporalis muscle, branches of the facial nerve, or the superficial temporal artery, which decreases operative exposure time when compared with a typical bifrontal craniotomy or pterional craniotomy.[15,21,26] An eyebrow incision eliminates the need for a hair shave and is easily hidden by the eyebrow, which decreases the psychological impact of surgery. If additional exposure is needed, the craniotomy can be expanded with an orbital rim osteotomy, medial supraorbital craniotomy, or conversion to a standard pterional craniotomy. Complications associated with the supraorbital approach include transient anesthesia over the frontal part of the scalp or transient frontalis muscle palsy.[15,16,21,26] Less common are CSF leaks and sinus fistula.[21] Avoiding the frontalis nerve is important for good cosmetic results. The course of the frontalis nerve can be plotted on the skin as a line starting from a point 0.5 cm below the tragus and passing 1.5 cm above the lateral extremity of the eyebrow.[58] Positioning is in the supine position with the head slightly rotated and extended to orient the surgical corridor vertically toward the lesion. This allows the frontal lobe to fall away from the floor of the anterior cranial fossa. An eyebrow incision can be made in the superior aspect of the eyebrow from the supraorbital notch to the lateral eyebrow. The pericranium is incised and raised as a separate flap, exposing the orbital rim and keyhole. A burr hole is then made in the keyhole, the underlying dura dissected free, and a craniotomy flap opened just lateral to the superior temporal line. The inner table of the frontal bone is then drilled flush with the orbital roof to flatten the exposure. Careful attention to the preoperative bony anatomy should be made and, if possible, avoiding the frontal sinus is recommended. The dura can then be opened as a flap based inferiorly. Intracranially, one priority is to open the arachnoid of the sylvian fissure and the olfactory and suprasellar cisterns for CSF drainage to create enough room for brain retraction and surgical manipulation.

Supraglabellar Approach

The supraglabellar approach is very similar to the supraorbital approach but allows a midline exposure to the base of the frontal fossa. The skin incision is made through a forehead skin crease, between supraorbital foramina laterally.[57] The craniotomy is performed with a craniotome between supraorbital foramina laterally, which then removes the frontal bone.[57] When accessing the frontal sinus with either the supraglabellar or the supraorbital approach, care must be given to prevent a posterior sinus tract or CSF leak. This is prevented by stripping the mucosa layer from the sinus and then filling it with fat or muscle at the end of the surgery. Once the dura is opened, the falx cerebri and the anterior tip of the superior sagittal sinus can be ligated.[57]

The visualization that each of the corridors and approaches described above can be achieved with an operating microscope; however, it can be much further increased by the use of straight and angled endoscopes. These will provide a panoramic view of the deeper structures. With the use of straight and angled lenses, visualization around nerves, vascular structures, and bony structures becomes possible and significantly better than a traditional microscope. Surgeries with only the use of an endoscopy are possible, especially with gradual learning and experience.

EQUIPMENT

To gain access and manipulate the tumor a special set of instruments for minimally invasive surgery should be accessible and prepared before surgery. A set of long and narrow instruments have been made for specific endonasal use and include irrigation devices, suction devices, drills, ultrasonic debriders, osteotomes, rongeurs, scissors, and cautery devices. The bipolar devices should have a range of angled tips to allow for easier coagulation through small narrow channels.[28] Likewise, the suction devices should also have a range of lengths, diameters, and angled tips to allow for access and evacuation of tumor. Neuronavigation and, possibly, intraoperative fluoroscopy should be available before starting each case. For surgical visualization, an operating microscope and/or endoscope setup should also be accessible. Two or more video screens in the room are also needed so that the remainder of the operating room team has an accurate knowledge of the surgical course.

Endoscopic Equipment

The rigid endoscope rod lens telescopes developed in the 1950s by Harold Hopkins, a professor of applied optical physics, improved the picture quality considerably.[7] This was then complimented by the fiberoptic cold-light light source by Karl Storz.[59] Current endoscopes are available through several companies come with varying sizes and lengths of shafts and lens angles. The angles range from 0° to 30°, 70°, and even 110°, and allow the surgeon to view all angles from the tip of the endoscope. Typically, the entire procedure is performed with a 0° endoscope. A bright xenon white light source and high-definition image system is necessary for adequate visualization. Endoscopes are reusable and provide excellent visual quality; however, owing to their rigidity and size, they often are difficult to maneuver. The physical positioning of the instruments and the two surgeons' four hands requires training and cannot be underestimated as an essential part of the case. Typically, the operating surgeon will need a cosurgeon to control the endoscope and prevent obstructing dissection instruments while maintaining adequate visualization (**Fig. 6**). Another method is to use a device to immobilize the endoscope, which allows the surgeons' hands to be freed for other instruments. However, for anterior skull base lesions and transplanum approaches, this is not preferred because dynamic control is needed for vascular control in bloody fields. For the two-surgeon technique, a binostril approach is used with one surgeon on each side of the patient or on one side of the patient (**Fig. 7**). Endoscopes and relevant instruments can be registered to a frameless neuronavigation system, which allows identification of the tip of the instrument in virtual space. To prevent the endoscope lens from becoming obscured by blood, a sheath over the endoscope that provides intermittent irrigation and cleaning is used. A 4 mm endoscope is used in adults, which allows passage of two to three more instruments for dissection or cauterization. Cautery must be available. The authors have had limited success with currently available, specially designed endoscopic pistol-grip bipolars and, typically, we use extended standard bayonet bipolars with straight or angled tips to reach the skull

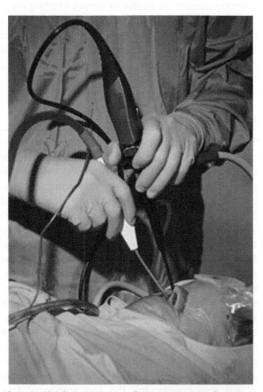

Fig. 6. Single-surgeon endoscope manipulation. A single surgeon working on the patient's right can hold the endoscope in the left hand atop the right naris and the surgical instrument in the right hand at the base of the right naris.

base. The typical instruments available for passage include various dissectors, suction freers, forceps, scissors, balloon dilation catheters, extended monopolar and bipolar cautery, CUSA debrider, microdebrider, and a CO_2 laser handpiece.

PREOPERATIVE CONSIDERATIONS

Any patient with a skull base lesion will need preoperative imaging. This consists of MRI of the brain and skull base. For lesions of the sella, high-quality pituitary or sellar protocol MRI is also performed. The internal carotid arteries, cavernous sinus, and anterior cerebral arteries should be evaluated for tumor encasement. Extension of tumor along the dura should be evaluated. The position of tumor in relation to cranial nerves should be evaluated because tumors that extend beyond functional cranial nerves, typically, should not be crossed with an endoscopic approach.[28] In some patients, fusing preoperative CT and MRI scans can allow better understanding of the correlation of the bony skull base and soft tissues. Also, special attention to the anatomy of the sinuses, especially in respect to septations, bony curvatures, and prior surgical openings, are helpful in identifying midline structures during surgery. Aeration of the posterior ethmoid cells above the sphenoid sinus, called Onodi cells, can lead to unrecognized exposure and injury of the optic nerve. A history of use, radiation therapy, or nasal-septal surgery may limit the use of the nasal septal flap and require an alternate flap (ie, turbinate or pericranial).

In all cases, provisions need to be made for the possibility of conversion of the minimally invasive approach to an open approach. Sometimes this will play a role into the positioning and prepping of the patient.

Some patients with anterior skull base lesions may be complicated with other underlying symptoms. Specifically, patients with endocrine abnormalities—typically, pituitary lesions or craniopharyngiomas—must be carefully evaluated for pituitary hypofunction and will need hormone replacement before surgery. Stress-dose steroids are most critically needed for patients whose tumors may cause adrenal insufficiency from damage to the pituitary gland. Patients with tumors whose resection requires work around the suprasellar cistern or pituitary gland are also at risk for perioperative diabetes insipidus and, therefore, must undergo postoperative monitoring for large volumes of dilute urine. Finally, preoperative testing should include evaluation of electrolytes and glucose.

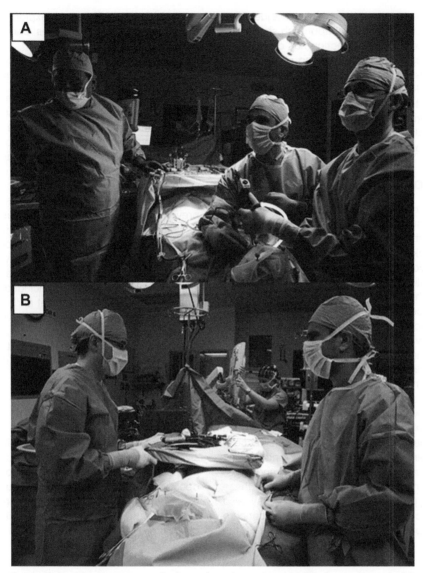

Fig. 7. Binostril approach with two surgeons. Endoscopic endonasal surgery can be performed with two surgeons working together: (*A*) with one surgeon on each side and the scope-holding surgeon on the right or (*B*) with both surgeons on the patient's right and the scope-holding surgeon up top.

PERIOPERATIVE CONSIDERATIONS

All patients undergoing anterior skull base procedure are under general anesthesia, which allows for strict control of blood pressure and intracranial pressure. During the surgery many of the structures of the anterior skull base are highly vascularized and, therefore, a lower or normal systolic blood pressure is recommended. Pretreatment with vasoconstricting agent to the mucosal layers can also help reduce bleeding in the corridors; however, monitoring the blood pressure during this application is imperative because of the potential for a systemic response. Finally, reducing

the positive end-expiratory pressure can help reduce venous pressure and bleeding. Leaving the head slightly elevated during surgery can reduce venous pressure and bleeding intraoperatively. At the completion of the surgical case, the field should be inspected again for bleeding. After the dural closing, a Valsalva maneuver is used to increase intrathoracic pressures, which would elicit a CSF leak if present.

Preoperative antibiotics are chosen to cover sinus bacteria and prevent meningeal bacteria. Ceftriaxone or cefepime is recommended.[60] Vancomycin and aztreonam can be administered to β-lactam–allergic patients.[60] If sinusitis is identified preoperatively, an intradural approach should not be undertaken until the infection has cleared.[61] If CSF is noticed during surgery and postoperative packing is used, postoperative antibiotics continue until the packing is removed.[60] Anticonvulsants are typically not dosed. A lumbar drain is typically placed when a CSF leaks is planned or identified. At the conclusion of surgery, mask ventilation is avoided to prevent tension pneumocephalus.

PATIENT POSITIONING AND ROOM SETUP

For the procedures associated with the approaches listed above, the patient is lying in the supine position with the head slightly extended and the neck slightly flexed. The head is immobilized in a rigid Mayfield or a semirigid gel doughnut. Horizontal alignment is critical to ensure the correct trajectory throughout the case. For fully endoscopic procedures, the room setup will include multiple pieces of equipment, including the endoscope, the video screens, Mayfield clamps, arms to secure the endoscope, neuroimaging devices, and irrigation equipment. The positioning of the surgeon, scrub technologist, and the neuroanesthesiologist becomes critical. One recommended setup is shown in **Fig. 8**. A thorough check before prepping the patient should be completed because the neuroanesthesiologist may have limited access to the patient, especially their face and airway, during the case. Typically, arterial lines and large-bore intravenous catheters are indicated for these intracranial procedures. The surgeon may also consider a central venous line if there is concern of a possible air embolus, for instance if the

cavernous sinus is likely to be explored. Reinforced endotracheal intubation tubes can be used to prevent kinking.

TUMOR RESECTION

Once the tumor is visualized, before resection, attention must be paid to the blood supply. Coagulation of the arterial supply can be followed by tumor debulking. Debulking allows for collapse of the tumor and easier manipulation and dissection. One method for tumor resection is using a two-suction technique in which gentle countertraction facilitates sharp extracapsular dissection. This prevents tearing and minimizes vascular injury because no grasping forceps is used.[49] This method is alternated with intratumor debulking. Tumor removal en bloc versus in layers was not shown to have a significant difference in outcome, in one series.[62] This series concluded that tumors with minimal dural involvement and minimal local invasion can be treated effectively with minimally invasive transnasal approaches.[63] In all malignant skull base tumors, it is recommend to remove as much tumor as possible, to remove a dural margin, and to remove all of the intracranial extension to achieve negative margins.

SKULL BASE RECONSTRUCTION

One of the greatest challenges of minimally invasive anterior cranial base surgery is to consistently provide closure of dural defects to prevent postoperative CSF leaks, pneumocephalus, and infection. There are several types of closures available, but these are limited owing to the availability of localized vascularized flaps. Other options for

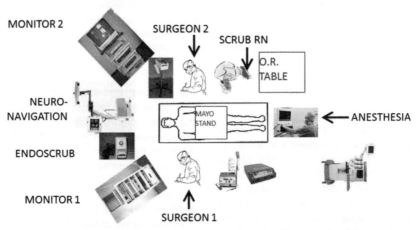

Fig. 8. Endoscopic room setup. The operating room for an endoscopic endonasal skull base surgery can be setup with the patient's head positioned away from anesthesia using an extended endotracheal tube. At the head of the patient, neuronavigation can be positioned in between two monitors, which allow the two surgeons to view the operation while working across from each other.

repair include microvascular free flap, pericranial scalp flap, synthetic dural substitute, suturable dural substitute, fat graft packing of the sphenoid sinus, and nasal packing with balloon catheters. For instance, at the authors' institution, openings for routine pituitary gland tumor resection are closed with devascularized tissue (free tissue fat graft and/or DuraGen).

Initially, in one large series of 800 cases closed using a variety of methods, the documented rate of postoperative CSF leak after endonasal endoscopic endonasal skull base surgery was 15.9%.[64] Other investigators report postoperative CSF leaks in up to 30% to 58% of their patients.[22,31,65,66] The current advantage of large craniofacial open techniques is the use of vascular pedicle flaps and suturing techniques that can provide a watertight seal and result in a postoperative CSF leak rate of less than 2%.[63] With minimally invasive approaches, the use of an NSF has been reported to significantly decrease postoperative CSF leak rates from 20% to less than 5% in multiple series,[64,67,68] results closer to those achieved with open approaches. The NSF has been based on a large posterior pedicle, which includes the nasoseptal artery, a branch of the posterior septal artery.[67] The addition of the pedicle originating near the sphenopalatine foramen clearly defines the arterial supply, allows harvest of large flaps composed of nearly the entire septal mucosa, and allows rotation of the flap in the posterior, superior, inferior, or lateral plane.[28] If prepared carefully during the opening of the procedure, this flap will be large enough to cover large dural defects from the frontal sinus to the sella. In a series at the authors' institution, 28 patients had 32 NSFs (either unilateral or bilateral) raised over 14 months; no cases of CSF leak or meningitis were noted with an average follow-up time of 8 months.[67] In select cases in which an NSF is unavailable, a middle or inferior turbinate flap can be used. In some cases, a bicoronal approach with pericranial flap is used and passed through a hole created in the nasal dorsum.

NSF PREPARATION

Several studies give evidence that the NSF decreases CSF leak rates postoperatively; therefore, the authors recommend NSFs for all large dural defects. At the beginning of the operation, an NSF is harvested as a mucoperichondrial flap based on the posterior nasoseptal artery, with incisions as described in a previous report.[67] After the mucosa is dissected off the sphenoid wall, a pedicle of mucosa from the sphenoid ostia to choanae and taken back to the level of the sphenopalatine foramen.[67] At the end of the case, once hemostasis is achieved, the exposed brain is covered with a synthetic dural substitute, such as DuraGen, and the edges are tucked intradurally.[61] Fat grafts can sometimes be used to cover the fascia and are in contact with the surrounding bone. The surface of the fat graft is covered with a cellulose material, Surgicel (Ethicon, Inc, Somerville, NJ, USA), to form an adherent crust.[61] The fat is then held in place with a fibrin sealant (Confluent Surgical, Inc, Waltham, MA, USA). Then the NSF is laid over it and secured with DuraSeal (Confluent Surgical Inc, Waltham, MA, USA). Careful attention should be made to ensure the NSF is oriented properly; the periosteal surface of flap must contact denuded walls of sinonasal tract (Video 2). Septal splints are placed over denuded septal cartilage and bone and left in place for 3 to 4 weeks.[67] Finally, gel foam (Pharmacia & Upjohn, Kalamazoo, MI, USA) covers the wound and a Foley balloon catheter (F12–14) crosses the nasopharynx posterior to the nasal septum before inflation with saline.[61] Two Merocel sponges are often used underneath the balloon.[67] A lumbar drain may be left in place for 3 to 5 days draining 10 to 20 cc/h, depending on the size and nature of the dural defect. The balloon is removed at 3 to 5 days and the Merocel sponges, when present, are removed at 10 days.[67] Also, the authors recommend no positive pressure ventilation for 3 days if there was no intraoperative CSF leak and for 1 month if there was an intraoperative CSF leak.

A special population of patients, characteristically obese, middle-aged women with elevated CSF pressures following repair, have an increased risk of postoperative CSF leak.[61] Patients who suffer from coughing or gagging during emergence from anesthesia, obstructive sleep apnea, morbid obesity, or excessive nose blowing cause elevated CSF pressure that also increases the risk of CSF leak.[61] Despite initial success, such patients remain at risk for recurrent CSF leaks months to years following repair. One helpful adjunct in patients who are at risk for CSF leak is to place a subarachnoid lumbar drain to allow CSF diversion, lower intracranial pressures, and allow healing of the nasal flap.[61] Overdrainage should be avoided because this creates a negative intracranial pressure (ie, suction effect) that may result in pneumocephalus and promote bacterial contamination of the CSF with resultant meningitis.[69]

POSTOPERATIVE CARE

Following surgery, patients with intracranial extension of tumor may benefit from a brief intensive care unit stay. Strict blood pressure control and neurologic examinations are carefully monitored.

A clinician should be aware of the possibility of postoperative diabetes insipidus occurring. Daily sodium levels and in-outs should be monitored. A postoperative MRI should be obtained before 48 hours. This will serve as a baseline MRI and assist the team in determining if further adjuvant radiation or chemotherapy is needed and where. Adjuvant therapy is specific for tumor type, histology, and quantity of residual tumor remaining.

Postoperatively, a clinician must also follow the patient closely and evaluate for CSF leak. Diagnosis of CSF leak in the postoperative patient can be challenging. The clinician should start by examining the patient for a CSF leak by asking them to lean forward for a period of time to elicit a leak. However, this is difficult if the nasal packing is in place. A postoperative CSF leak can confirmed with a beta-2 transferrin test. However, if nasal leakage is uncertain to be CSF, the presence of CSF in the nasal cavity at the time of surgery may confuse interpretation of this test. Subsequently, identifying where the leak is coming from is needed to plan the repair. Starting with a thorough endoscopic examination of the nasal cavity may reveal the site of the leak.[69] In addition, a high resolution CT scan of the sinuses with contrast may prove useful.[69] If a sizable defect is noted, a follow-up MRI may be indicated to investigate a possible meningocele or encephalocele. The T2 imaging on MRI can often identify the presence of a leak. If the concern is high or findings inconclusive, intrathecal injection of contrast materials in combination of high-resolution bone coronal CT scan and/or radioactive tracers can confirm a CSF leak and identify the site of origin.[69] Typically, CSF leak from an apparent defect in the primary closure should be repaired in the operating room.

SURGICAL OUTCOMES

Malignant pathologic lesions located in the anterior skull base consist of rare tumors that often present in an aggressive invasive stage. Therefore, much of the literature on skull base malignancies, whether resection occurs via a minimally invasive approach or a larger craniofacial approach, is characterized by single-institution experiences with pooled results from a variety of tumor locations, histology, and treatment plans. Comparing treatment plans, tumor response, recurrence rate, and survival rates between studies to arrive at standard protocols can be challenging.

Several reviews attempt this comparison, although many have significant differences between the two patient cohorts, which make their results uncertain. In one review, multiple tumor types were evaluated and compared with open and minimal invasive approaches.[70] The results were notable for craniopharyngiomas, clival chordomas, esthesioneuroblastomas, and giant pituitary adenomas endonasal endoscopic approach resulting in higher rate of GTR for endoscopic approaches.[70] Open cranial procedures had a higher GTR for meningiomas.[70] CSF leaks, however, were higher in patients recovering from endoscopic surgery.[70] Interestingly, one study reviewing skull base meningiomas notes that the use of the endoscope allowed further visualization of tumor that a microscope could not see in 65% of patients.[30] GTR was noted in 76% cases and near total resection in the remaining 24%.[30] Another study in which minimally invasive technique was used for craniopharyngiomas reports 91% of patient received gross total or near total resection.[31] For chordomas GTR was reported in 66.7% in a series of 60 patients; however, this rate improved to 88.9% in the later years of the study, giving evidence the importance of experience with minimally invasive approaches.[50]

A literature review comparing only open transcranial versus transsphenoidal craniopharyngiomas showed that the endoscopic study had greater rate of total resection and improved postoperative visual outcome.[71] However the rate of CSF leak was higher in the endoscopic group (18%) versus in the transcranial group (3%).[71] Two smaller studies retrospectively reviewed the experience with endoscopic approaches to the suprasellar tumors through transtuberculum and transplanum sphenoidale approaches.[72,73] In these studies, the incidence of postoperative CSF rhinorrhea was 15% to 25%. This rate was decreased with the use of vascular flaps instead of mucosal free grafts. The rate of GTR was greater than 80%.

Another meta-analysis that reviewed 379 patients with esthesioneuroblastoma resulted in a Kaplan-Meier analysis that showed improved survival with endoscopic resection compared with open craniofacial resection (hazard ratio, 3.56; 95% CI, 1.61–7.91), with similar follow-up in the endoscopic and open groups (54.5 vs 51.0 months).[74]

Finally, in a review of over 800 endoscopic endonasal cases, the mortality rate was 0.9% and the rate of permanent neurologic deficit was 1.8%.[64] In total, these studies, although well short of Level 1 evidence, support the notion that minimally invasive approaches performed by experienced surgeons are safe and provide benefit with the correct patient selection.

PREVENTION OF COMPLICATIONS

In addition to CSF leak, another challenging complication during minimally invasive anterior skull based surgery is hemostasis.[28] One possibility to improve control in vascular tumors is to obtain an angiogram with embolization preoperatively. During surgery, attempting to ligate the tumor from the dural attachment quickly and ligate feeding ethmoidal arteries decreases heavy bleeding.[28] Hemostasis can also be eased by reducing high venous pressure by changing the patient's position and the ventilator settings. Another recommendation is to use a diamond drill tip, which acts with more hemostatic effect when removing bone.[28] If major vascular injury does occur during surgery, packing or clipping is typically used to bridge the patient to the neurovascular suite for angiogram and possible interventional repair. Using a micro-Doppler to identify vasculature structures—specifically, the position of the carotid—helps with navigation intraoperatively.

Postoperative infections, including bacterial meningitis, tend to have a low incidence of 1% to 2%.[60,61,64] This has been attributed to the use of perioperative antibiotics, frequent irrigation intraoperatively, careful reconstruction with vascularized flaps, and no need for nonbiodegradable materials left at the completion of the surgery.[61] Risk factors for infection include male sex, complex tumors, presence of an external ventricular drain or shunt, and postoperative CSF leak.[60]

Difficult Patients

Pediatric patients have smaller nares and allow less room for instrumentation. However, children over the age of 4 typically have enough room for these procedures.[61] Also patients with decreased sinus pneumatization, including pediatric patients, have more difficult anatomy to navigate intraoperatively. Neuronavigation is of the utmost importance for cases like these.[61]

SUMMARY

Application of instruments from endoscopic sinus surgery to skull base tumors has allowed neurosurgeons and otolaryngologist to perform minimally invasive resection of malignant tumors in the anterior skull base for the past decade. Minimally invasive approaches reduce the need for more extensive surgical approaches, which allows less soft tissue manipulation and brain tissue exposure, shorter recovery times, and offers a better cosmetic result. Surgical planning includes determining the target, entry point, and corridor with the least amount of vascular and neural manipulation. Not all tumors, given their size, invasion, and locations are amenable to these minimally invasive approaches; therefore, patient selection is critical. The use of minimally invasive

approaches, especially when coupled with endoscopy, is best when both neurosurgeon and otolaryngologist work and learn together while understanding their limitations. Minimally invasive anterior skull base approaches continue to gain acceptance as a safe and effective approach to remove malignant lesions. Further randomized, controlled studies are needed to investigate and confirm the many benefits this approach has to offer.

SUPPLEMENTARY DATA

Supplementary data related to this article can be found online at http://dx.doi.org/10.1016/j.nec.2012.08.001.

REFERENCES

1. El Gindi S. Neurosurgery in Egypt: past, present, and future-from pyramids to radiosurgery. Neurosurgery 2002;51:789.
2. Artico M, Pastore FS, Fraioli B, et al. The contribution of Davide Giordano (1864-1954) to pituitary surgery: the transglabellar-nasal approach. Neurosurgery 1998;42:909.
3. Liu JK, Cohen-Gadol AA, Laws ER Jr, et al. Harvey Cushing and Oskar Hirsch: early forefathers of modern transsphenoidal surgery. J Neurosurg 2005;103:1096.
4. Lanzino G, Laws ER Jr. Key personalities in the development and popularization of the transsphenoidal approach to pituitary tumors: an historical overview. Neurosurg Clin N Am 2003;14:1.
5. Maroon JC. Skull base surgery: past, present, and future trends. Neurosurg Focus 2005;19:E1.
6. Couldwell WT. Transsphenoidal and transcranial surgery for pituitary adenomas. J Neurooncol 2004; 69:237.
7. Abbott R. Neuroendoscopy: indications for its use. Surg Technol Int 1995;IV:393.
8. Pettorini BL, Tamburrini G. Two hundred years of endoscopic surgery: from Philipp Bozzini's cystoscope to paediatric endoscopic neurosurgery. Childs Nerv Syst 2007;23:723.
9. Gandhi CD, Christiano LD, Eloy JA, et al. The historical evolution of transsphenoidal surgery: facilitation by technological advances. Neurosurg Focus 2009; 27:E8.
10. Liu JK, Das K, Weiss MH, et al. The history and evolution of transsphenoidal surgery. J Neurosurg 2001; 95:1083.
11. Jankowski R, Auque J, Simon C, et al. Endoscopic pituitary tumor surgery. Laryngoscope 1992;102:198.
12. Sethi DS, Pillay PK. Endoscopic management of lesions of the sella turcica. J Laryngol Otol 1995; 109:956.

13. Kassam A, Snyderman CH, Mintz A, et al. Expanded endonasal approach: the rostrocaudal axis. Part I. Crista galli to the sella turcica. Neurosurg Focus 2005;19:E3.

14. Hadad G, Bassagasteguy L, Carrau RL, et al. A novel reconstructive technique after endoscopic expanded endonasal approaches: vascular pedicle nasoseptal flap. Laryngoscope 2006;116:1882.

15. Park HS, Park SK, Han YM. Microsurgical experience with supraorbital keyhole operations on anterior circulation aneurysms. J Korean Neurosurg Soc 2009;46:103.

16. Zhang MZ, Wang L, Zhang W, et al. The supraorbital keyhole approach with eyebrow incisions for treating lesions in the anterior fossa and sellar region. Chin Med J (Engl) 2004;117:323.

17. McArthur L. Asseptic surgical access to the pituitary body and its neighborhood. JAMA 1912; 58:2009.

18. Frazier CH. I. An approach to the hypophysis through the anterior cranial fossa. Ann Surg 1913; 57:145.

19. Jane JA, Park TS, Pobereskin LH, et al. The supraorbital approach: technical note. Neurosurgery 1982; 11:537.

20. van Lindert E, Perneczky A, Fries G, et al. The supraorbital keyhole approach to supratentorial aneurysms: concept and technique. Surg Neurol 1998;49:481.

21. Fernandes YB, Maitrot D, Kehrli P, et al. Supraorbital eyebrow approach to skull base lesions. Arq Neuropsiquiatr 2002;60:246.

22. Gardner PA, Kassam AB, Thomas A, et al. Endoscopic endonasal resection of anterior cranial base meningiomas. Neurosurgery 2008;63:36.

23. Ceylan S, Koc K, Anik I. Extended endoscopic transsphenoidal approach for tuberculum sellae meningiomas. Acta Neurochir (Wien) 2011;153:1.

24. de Divitiis E, Esposito F, Cappabianca P, et al. Tuberculum sellae meningiomas: high route or low route? A series of 51 consecutive cases. Neurosurgery 2008;62:556.

25. Wang Q, Lu XJ, Ji WY, et al. Visual outcome after extended endoscopic endonasal transsphenoidal surgery for tuberculum sellae meningiomas. World Neurosurg 2010;73:694.

26. Wongsirisuwan M. What is the better minimally invasive surgery in pituitary surgery: endoscopic endonasal transsphenoidal approach or keyhole supraorbital approach? J Med Assoc Thai 2011;94:888.

27. Schwartz TH, Fraser JF, Brown S, et al. Endoscopic cranial base surgery: classification of operative approaches. Neurosurgery 2008;62:991.

28. Snyderman CH, Pant H, Carrau RL, et al. What are the limits of endoscopic sinus surgery?: the expanded endonasal approach to the skull base. Keio J Med 2009;58:152.

29. Simpson D. The recurrence of intracranial meningiomas after surgical treatment. J Neurol Neurosurg Psychiatry 1957;20:22.

30. Schroeder HW, Hickmann AK, Baldauf J. Endoscope-assisted microsurgical resection of skull base meningiomas. Neurosurg Rev 2011;34:441.

31. Gardner PA, Kassam AB, Snyderman CH, et al. Outcomes following endoscopic, expanded endonasal resection of suprasellar craniopharyngiomas: a case series. J Neurosurg 2008;109:6.

32. Vrionis FD, Kienstra MA, Rivera M, et al. Malignant tumors of the anterior skull base. Cancer Control 2004;11:144.

33. Kadish S, Goodman M, Wang CC. Olfactory neuroblastoma. A clinical analysis of 17 cases. Cancer 1976;37:1571.

34. Kane AJ, Sughrue ME, Rutkowski MJ, et al. Posttreatment prognosis of patients with esthesioneuroblastoma. J Neurosurg 2010;113:340.

35. Folbe A, Herzallah I, Duvvuri U, et al. Endoscopic endonasal resection of esthesioneuroblastoma: a multicenter study. Am J Rhinol Allergy 2009;23:91.

36. Nicolai P, Battaglia P, Bignami M, et al. Endoscopic surgery for malignant tumors of the sinonasal tract and adjacent skull base: a 10-year experience. Am J Rhinol 2008;22:308.

37. Lund V, Howard DJ, Wei WI. Endoscopic resection of malignant tumors of the nose and sinuses. Am J Rhinol 2007;21:89.

38. Revenaugh PC, Seth R, Pavlovich JB, et al. Minimally invasive endoscopic resection of sinonasal undifferentiated carcinoma. Am J Otolaryngol 2011;32:464.

39. Reiersen DA, Pahilan ME, Devaiah AK. Meta-analysis of treatment outcomes for sinonasal undifferentiated carcinoma. Otolaryngol Head Neck Surg 2012;147:7.

40. Chen AM, Daly ME, El-Sayed I, et al. Patterns of failure after combined-modality approaches incorporating radiotherapy for sinonasal undifferentiated carcinoma of the head and neck. Int J Radiat Oncol Biol Phys 2008;70:338.

41. Menon S, Pai P, Sengar M, et al. Sinonasal malignancies with neuroendocrine differentiation: case series and review of literature. Indian J Pathol Microbiol 2010;53:28.

42. Weng CT, Chu PY, Liu MT, et al. Small cell carcinoma of the head and neck: a single institution's experience and review of the literature. J Otolaryngol Head Neck Surg 2008;37:788.

43. Fordice J, Kershaw C, El-Naggar A, et al. Adenoid cystic carcinoma of the head and neck: predictors of morbidity and mortality. Arch Otolaryngol Head Neck Surg 1999;125:149.

44. Ellington CL, Goodman M, Kono SA, et al. Adenoid cystic carcinoma of the head and neck: incidence and survival trends based on 1973-2007 surveillance,

epidemiology, and end results data. Cancer 2012; 118:4444–51.

45. Eibling DE, Janecka IP, Snyderman CH, et al. Meta-analysis of outcome in anterior skull base resection for squamous cell and undifferentiated carcinoma. Skull Base Surg 1993;3:123.

46. Ganly I, Patel SG, Singh B, et al. Craniofacial resection for malignant melanoma of the skull base: report of an international collaborative study. Arch Otolaryngol Head Neck Surg 2006;132:73.

47. Frank G, Sciarretta V, Calbucci F, et al. The endoscopic transnasal transsphenoidal approach for the treatment of cranial base chordomas and chondrosarcomas. Neurosurgery 2006;59:ONS50.

48. Colli BO, Al-Mefty O. Chordomas of the skull base: follow-up review and prognostic factors. Neurosurg Focus 2001;10:E1.

49. Stippler M, Gardner PA, Snyderman CH, et al. Endoscopic endonasal approach for clival chordomas. Neurosurgery 2009;64:268.

50. Koutourousiou M, Gardner PA, Tormenti MJ, et al. Endoscopic endonasal approach for resection of skull base chordomas: outcomes and learning curve. Neurosurgery 2012;71(3):614–25.

51. Sen C, Triana AI, Berglind N, et al. Clival chordomas: clinical management, results, and complications in 71 patients. J Neurosurg 2010;113:1059.

52. Crockard HA, Steel T, Plowman N, et al. A multidisciplinary team approach to skull base chordomas. J Neurosurg 2001;95:175.

53. Gay E, Sekhar LN, Rubinstein E, et al. Chordomas and chondrosarcomas of the cranial base: results and follow-up of 60 patients. Neurosurgery 1995; 36:887.

54. Tzortzidis F, Elahi F, Wright D, et al. Patient outcome at long-term follow-up after aggressive microsurgical resection of cranial base chordomas. Neurosurgery 2006;59:230.

55. Pirris SM, Pollack IF, Snyderman CH, et al. Corridor surgery: the current paradigm for skull base surgery. Childs Nerv Syst 2007;23:377.

56. Solares CA, Fakhri S, Batra PS, et al. Transnasal endoscopic resection of lesions of the clivus: a preliminary report. Laryngoscope 2005;115:1917.

57. Hammad O, Ali A. Mini craniotomy for anterior skull base lesions. EJNS 2006;21:103.

58. Pitanguy I, Ramos AS. The frontal branch of the facial nerve: the importance of its variations in face lifting. Plast Reconstr Surg 1966;38:352.

59. Fuchs GJ. Milestones in endoscope design for minimally invasive urologic surgery: the sentinel role of a pioneer. Surg Endosc 2006;20(Suppl 2):S493.

60. Kono Y, Prevedello DM, Snyderman CH, et al. One thousand endoscopic skull base surgical procedures demystifying the infection potential: incidence and description of postoperative meningitis and brain abscesses. Infect Control Hosp Epidemiol 2011;32:77.

61. Snyderman CH, Kassam AB, Carrau R, et al. Endoscopic reconstruction of cranial base defects following endonasal skull base surgery. Skull Base 2007;17:73.

62. Soler ZM, Smith TL. Endoscopic versus open craniofacial resection of esthesioneuroblastoma: what is the evidence? Laryngoscope 2012;122:244.

63. Zimmer LA, Theodosopoulos PV. Anterior skull base surgery: open versus endoscopic. Curr Opin Otolaryngol Head Neck Surg 2009;17:75.

64. Kassam AB, Prevedello DM, Carrau RL, et al. Endoscopic endonasal skull base surgery: analysis of complications in the authors' initial 800 patients. J Neurosurg 2011;114:1544.

65. Feiz-Erfan I, Han PP, Spetzler RF, et al. The radical transbasal approach for resection of anterior and midline skull base lesions. J Neurosurg 2005;103:485.

66. Gardner PA, Prevedello DM, Kassam AB, et al. The evolution of the endonasal approach for craniopharyngiomas. J Neurosurg 2008;108:1043.

67. El-Sayed IH, Roediger FC, Goldberg AN, et al. Endoscopic reconstruction of skull base defects with the nasal septal flap. Skull Base 2008;18:385.

68. Kassam AB, Thomas A, Carrau RL, et al. Endoscopic reconstruction of the cranial base using a pedicled nasoseptal flap. Neurosurgery 2008;63:ONS44.

69. Carrau RL, Snyderman CH, Kassam AB. The management of cerebrospinal fluid leaks in patients at risk for high-pressure hydrocephalus. Laryngoscope 2005;115:205.

70. Komotar RJ, Starke RM, Raper DM, et al. Endoscopic skull base surgery: a comprehensive comparison with open transcranial approaches. Br J Neurosurg 2012;77(2):329–41.

71. Komotar RJ, Starke RM, Raper DM, et al. Endoscopic endonasal compared with microscopic transsphenoidal and open transcranial resection of craniopharyngiomas. World Neurosurg 2012; 77:329.

72. de Divitiis E, Cavallo LM, Esposito F, et al. Extended endoscopic transsphenoidal approach for tuberculum sellae meningiomas. Neurosurgery 2007;61:229.

73. Stamm AC, Vellutini E, Harvey RJ, et al. Endoscopic transnasal craniotomy and the resection of craniopharyngioma. Laryngoscope 2008;118:1142.

74. Devaiah AK, Andreoli MT. Treatment of esthesioneuroblastoma: a 16-year meta-analysis of 361 patients. Laryngoscope 2009;119:1412.

Sinonasal Carcinomas
Epidemiology, Pathology, and Management

Stephan K. Haerle, MD[a],
Patrick J. Gullane, CM, MB, FRCSC[a],*,
Ian J. Witterick, MD, MSc, FRCSC[a], Christian Zweifel, MD[b],
Fred Gentili, MD, MSc, FRCSC[b]

KEYWORDS

- Sinonasal carcinoma • Skull base • Epidemiology • Pathology • Management

KEY POINTS

- Sinonasal malignancies are uncommon neoplasms, and in most cases present in an advanced stage of disease.
- Exact staging necessitates a clinical and endoscopic examination with biopsy and imaging.
- Tumor resection using an open or endoscopic approach is usually considered as the first treatment option.
- In general, sinonasal carcinomas are radiosensitive and, therefore, adjuvant or neoadjuvant radiation treatment may be indicated in advanced disease.
- Multidisciplinary surgical and medical oncologic approaches, which include ablation and reconstruction, have enhanced the survival outcome over the past few decades.

INTRODUCTION

Sinonasal carcinomas are uncommon neoplasms that account for approximately 3% to 5% of all upper respiratory tract malignancies. Sinonasal malignancies in most cases do not cause early symptoms and present in an advanced stage of disease. In general, sinonasal carcinomas are radiosensitive; therefore, adjuvant or neoadjuvant radiation treatment may be indicated in advanced disease. Multidisciplinary surgical and medical oncologic approaches, which include ablation and reconstruction, have enhanced the survival outcome over the past few decades.

Epidemiology

Sinonasal carcinomas are uncommon malignancies, with an estimated incidence in the United States of 0.556 cases per 100,000 population.[1] This figure represents approximately 0.2% of all cancers and 3% to 5% of cancers in the upper aerodigestive tract.[2–4] The majority of published reports have identified the maxillary sinus to be the most common primary site.[4–8] Other studies have reported this to be the nasal cavity.[1,9] Because sinonasal malignancies often present in an advanced stage, the true identification of the site of origin may be difficult. Primary malignancy of the frontal sinus is uncommon, and those arising in the sphenoid sinus are rare.[10,11]

[a] Department of Otolaryngology – Head and Neck Surgery, Toronto General Hospital, University Health Network, 200 Elizabeth Street, Toronto, Ontario M5G 2C4, Canada; [b] Division of Neurosurgery, Toronto General Hospital, University Health Network, 399 Bathurst Street, Toronto, Ontario M5T 2S8, Canada
* Corresponding author. Department of Otolaryngology – Head and Neck Surgery, University of Toronto, University Health Network/Toronto General Hospital, 200 Elizabeth Street, Room 8N-877, Toronto, Ontario M5G 2C4, Canada.
E-mail address: Patrick.gullane@uhn.ca

Neurosurg Clin N Am 24 (2013) 39–49
http://dx.doi.org/10.1016/j.nec.2012.08.004

Sinonasal carcinomas arise most often during the sixth decade of life with a male to female ratio of approximately 2:1. A recent study of population-based data (Surveillance, Epidemiology, and End Results [SEER]) included more than 6000 patients, and reported a decrease in the incidence of sinonasal cancer in men while remaining stable among women.[1] These findings reflect changing demographics and the socioeconomic developments seen also in other head and neck cancers.[12]

Risk Factors

Several occupational risk factors have been reported. Adenocarcinomas have been associated with hardwood dust exposure, chrome pigment, clothing, and leather, whereas squamous cell carcinoma (SCC) has been linked with nickel, soft wood dust, radium, mustard gas, and asbestos.[13–15] Occupational exposures such as those involving the use of formaldehyde have been shown to increase the risk of both adenocarcinoma and SCC.[15] Unlike other head and neck cancers, cigarette smoking and alcohol have less impact on the development of sinonasal carcinoma.

More recently, human papilloma virus (HPV) has also been associated with the malignant transformation of inverted papilloma and SCC.[16,17] Similar to HPV-associated SCC of the oropharynx, tumors in the sinonasal region that are HPV positive have a better treatment outcome.[18]

PATHOLOGY
Anatomy

The nasal cavity and the paranasal sinuses are in close proximity to many vital structures that can be involved by the contiguous spread of tumor. In addition, the paranasal sinuses have lymphatic and venous drainage pathways, which provide additional routes of spread intracranially. The skull base forms the floor of the cranial cavity and separates the brain from a variety of other important facial structures. The bony architecture of the skull base consists of the ethmoid, sphenoid, occipital, paired frontal, and parietal bones. Three regions can be differentiated: the anterior, middle, and posterior cranial fossae. In the case of sinonasal malignancy, the anterior skull base is the most commonly affected region. Thus, exact anatomic knowledge of the paranasal sinuses and anterior skull base is important for the treatment of sinonasal malignancies.

Staging

Because of late presentation, the diagnosis of malignant sinonasal tumors in patients often occurs in the later stages, so it is difficult to determine the exact site of tumor origin. The first staging system was described by Ohngren, and was based on resectability criteria established by the extension of the tumor with respect to Ohngren's line (connecting the angle of the mandible with the medial canthus).[19] Since then, a variety of classification systems have been published, including the seventh TNM classification system by the American Joint Committee on Cancer (AJCC).[20] There is a recognized correlation between tumor extension and treatment outcome. A review by the International Collaborative Group demonstrated that the histology, grade, intracranial extent, and status of surgical margins were independent predictors of treatment outcome.[21] The different staging systems for olfactory neuroblastoma are separately described in the relevant section of this article.

HISTOLOGIC SUBTYPES

Sinonasal carcinomas present with a variation of histologic heterogeneity in tumor type. The sinonasal tract and skull base is a region with the greatest histologic diversity in the body, and this

---

Box 1
Malignant sinonasal tumors

- Epithelial
  - Squamous cell carcinoma
  - Adenocarcinoma
  - Salivary-gland type tumors
    - Adenoid cystic carcinoma
    - Mucoepidermoid carcinoma
    - Acinic cell carcinoma
  - Sinonasal undifferentiated carcinoma
- Neuroectodermal
  - Melanoma
  - Olfactory neuroblastoma
- Neuroendocrine
  - Sinonasal neuroendocrine carcinoma
- Soft-tissue tumors
- Borderline and low malignant potential tumors of soft tissue
- Malignant tumors of bone and cartilage
- Hematolymphoid tumors
- Neuroectodermal tumors
- Germ cell tumors
- Secondary tumors

is reflected in the extensive disorder classification list compiled by the World Health Organization (WHO).[22,23] The major malignant subtypes are presented in **Box 1**. This article reviews the more common epithelial, neuroectodermal, and neuroendocrine type tumors. There are other more rare malignancies (eg, bone or soft-tissue tumors) that may also occur.

Squamous Cell Carcinoma

The most commonly encountered malignant neoplasms of the sinonasal tract are the keratinizing and nonkeratinizing types of SCC.[24] In 1% to 7% of all cases, SCC is seen in association with inverted papilloma.[25,26] SCC of the nasal cavity arises in the paranasal sinuses more frequently than in the nasal cavity.[27] The majority of SCC of the paranasal sinuses are keratinizing and nonkeratinizing lesions, with the undifferentiated type being less frequent. The latter subtype shows a more rapid course of growth. Similar to other locations in the head and neck, the basaloid variant of SCC has a more aggressive biological behavior.[28]

Early-stage disease (T1/T2) arising from the nasal cavity can be effectively managed by single-modality treatment (surgery or radiotherapy), whereas advanced-stage disease (T3/T4) requires a combined approach. SCC of the paranasal sinuses is often diagnosed at a late stage, and regional spread to the lymph nodes may be present.[29,30] Therefore elective treatment of the neck may be considered, especially when the SCC of the paranasal sinuses has invaded the overlaying soft tissue or adjacent bony structures.[31] The 5-year survival rates reported for SCC of the paranasal sinuses and the nasal cavity range from 40% to 70%.[6,32]

Adenocarcinoma

Adenocarcinoma represents the third most common malignancy in the sinonasal tract, after SCC and adenoid cystic carcinoma. It accounts for approximately 15% of all sinonasal cancers and is associated with certain risk factors.[2] Adenocarcinoma is male dominant and presents most frequently in the ethmoid sinuses. This malignancy is divided into a salivary-gland and non–salivary-gland type.[33,34] The latter is further separated into intestinal and nonintestinal types. Subclassifications of the intestinal type include papillary, colonic, solid, mucinous, or mixed, and the nonintestinal types are classified as either low or high grade. Intestinal-type carcinomas are generally aggressive with a local recurrence rate of up to 50%, lymphatic spread in 10%, and a distant metastasis rate of 20%. Low-grade nonintestinal

adenocarcinomas most frequently occur in the ethmoid cells, and the 5-year survival rate is up to 85%. The high-grade nonintestinal adenocarcinomas are more commonly found in the maxillary sinus and have a very poor prognosis (3-year survival approximately 20%).[2] The majority of the adenocarcinomas arise from the mucoserous glands while the remainder originates in the respiratory epithelium.[35]

Many patients with adenocarcinomas are effectively treated with radiotherapy. However, surgical excision followed by radiotherapy is favored in many centers throughout the world. An open radical craniofacial resection is often warranted, and in many cases adjuvant radiotherapy needs to be scheduled because the disease is usually recognized in an advanced stage.[36] In carefully selected patients, a curative endoscopic approach may be considered. Another method of treatment involves surgical debulking via an endoscopic or open approach in combination with repeated topical chemotherapy (5-fluorouracil). Radiotherapy in this case is only given in cases of local recurrence.[37] Ten-year survival rates are reported to exceed 70%.[36,37]

Adenoid Cystic Carcinoma

Adenoid cystic carcinoma (ACC) is the second most common tumor of the nasal cavity and paranasal sinuses, and accounts for approximately 10% of all non-SCC in the head and neck region and 15% of all salivary-gland cancers.[38–40] It arises more frequently in minor salivary glands than in all major salivary glands combined. Histologically, ACC exhibits 3 different subtypes based on the tumor architecture: cribriform, tubular, and solid. The cribriform pattern with its familiar stromal architecture is the most common. The tubular pattern, with a more typical glandular formation, has the best prognosis, and the less common solid pattern has the worst outcome. ACC in general is a slow-growing neoplasm, and recurrences often develop 10 to 20 years after initial treatment. ACC has a propensity for perineural spread and intracranial extension, reflecting the challenges of treating ACC and high morbidity. The most frequently involved nerves are the maxillary, mandibular, and vidian nerves. Because negative surgical resection margins may be difficult to achieve, ACC of the sinonasal tract has a poor prognosis.[39,41] Lymphatic spread to regional lymph nodes is uncommon and accounts for 10% to 30% of patients, whereas distant hematogenous spread is more frequent, with an average incidence of 40%.[42,43] The propensity for distant spread correlates with the stage at presentation, and the most commonly affected distant sites are the lungs and long bones.

Surgical treatment with negative surgical margins is the gold standard for treating ACC. Postoperative radiation is used to achieve better local control, although the association with increasing survival remains controversial.[44,45] The role of systemic therapy is yet to be defined, although it has been shown to benefit some patients with recurrent, metastatic, and/or unresectable disease. Systemic therapy mainly consists of cisplatin alone or in combination with other agents (eg, doxorubicin, 5-fluorouracil), and the reported response rates to chemotherapy have been inconsistent and remain less than 20%.[46]

Mucoepidermoid Carcinoma

Mucoepidermoid carcinoma (MEC) of the sinonasal tract is the second most common sinonasal salivary-gland type of malignancy after ACC. Differential diagnoses include adenosquamous carcinoma, adenocarcinoma, and necrotizing sialometaplasia. Overall, MEC accounts for fewer than 0.1% of all malignant sinonasal tract neoplasms, with no gender difference in disease prevalence.[47] MEC are histologically graded as low, intermediate, or high grade, with the latter having the worst prognosis. Clinical symptoms are nonspecific and usually present over a period of months. Invasive growth in MEC is common and recurrence is seen in approximately one-third of patients, usually within 2 years.[47] Surgery with the achievement of clear margins is the treatment of choice. Adjuvant radiotherapy in cases of positive margins is suggested to improve survival to the same level as that in patients with negative surgical margins. In cases of a high-grade tumor with negative resection margins, adjuvant radiotherapy is usually considered because of the aggressiveness of these tumors. Loh and colleagues[48] reported that disease-free survival for MEC in the nasal cavity was poorer than that for MEC in the oral cavity. MEC was associated with a greater tendency for local recurrences, which may be due to the incomplete tumor resection resulting from anatomic limitations.[48]

Acinic Cell Carcinoma

Acinic cell carcinoma is a low-grade malignant epithelial salivary-gland malignancy presenting very rarely in the sinonasal tract. Acinic cell carcinomas are most commonly found in the fifth and sixth decades of life, but are also reported in children.[49,50] There is no gender preference in the occurrence of these sinonasal tumors. Acinic cell carcinoma is believed to arise from the intercalated duct reserve cells.[49] Different grading systems and prognosis-related factors are described, but these studies are limited by small sample sizes and mainly concern major salivary glands outside the sinonasal tract. Laskawi and colleagues[51] found that histologically well-differentiated tumors in the parotid gland correlate with better prognosis than do poorly differentiated acinic cell carcinomas. There is a very low chance of nodal spread when the tumor originates in the sinonasal tract. The treatment of choice is surgical excision with adjuvant radiotherapy in patients with positive resection margins, perineural invasion, and/or lymphovascular invasion.[49] Similarly to ACC, patients with acinic cell carcinoma should be followed for long periods of time because metastases may occur many years after treatment.

Sinonasal Undifferentiated Carcinoma

Sinonasal undifferentiated carcinoma (SNUC) was first described by Frierson and colleagues[52] in 1986. SNUC is a very rare and aggressive malignancy that is hypothesized to be part of the spectrum of neuroendocrine carcinomas that include olfactory neuroblastoma, neuroendocrine carcinoma, and small cell carcinoma.[53] Usually it incorporates extensive tissue destruction and involvement of the orbit and anterior cranial fossa.[54] In general, light microscopy can differentiate between SNUC and other differential diagnoses such as olfactory neuroblastoma, lymphoma, rhabdomyosarcoma, and melanoma. In some cases, immunohistochemistry or electron microscopy is required to confirm the diagnosis. Differentiation between SNUC and olfactory neuroblastoma is important because the clinical behavior, prognosis, and treatment differ: olfactory neuroblastoma is generally slow growing with a better prognosis, whereas SNUC progresses more rapidly with a poor prognosis.[55] SNUC has been associated with Epstein-Barr virus; however, its role has not yet been confirmed.[55] The best treatment strategy for these tumors has yet to be defined. Some physicians have described preoperative chemotherapy followed by radiotherapy. In cases with no extensive intracranial involvement and without the presence of distant disease, a definitive surgical resection can be performed.[56] A recent meta-analysis of treatment outcomes for SNUC reported that treatment should include surgery, with radiation and/or chemotherapy as adjunctive treatments.[57] The role of induction chemotherapy in limiting the extent of surgery remains to be established.

Melanoma

Melanoma of the sinonasal tract is rare and accounts for only 1% of all melanomas.[58] The nasal cavity is the most commonly affected site, followed by the maxillary antrum and the ethmoid sinuses, and it usually occurs between the fifth and eighth decades of life.[59] Clinical examination can be challenging when the melanoma is amelanotic because the typical heavily pigmented polypoid or fleshy mass is absent. Several histologic subtypes are described: amelanotic small blue cell, pleomorphic, epithelioid, spindle cell, and myxoid. All of these subtypes show a high mitotic rate, vascular invasion, regression, and absence of tumor-infiltrating lymphocytes.[60] Usually the presence of melanin helps to confirm the diagnosis. However, in the absence of melanin, specific stains are used to differentiate mucosal melanoma from other diagnoses such as anaplastic carcinoma, lymphoma, and olfactory neuroblastoma. In general, the prognosis of patients diagnosed with sinonasal mucosal melanoma is poor, with an average 5-year actuarial survival rate of less than 15%.[59,61] Patients with lesions that present on the nasal septum tend to do better than those with lesions at other sites within the sinonasal tract.[62] Primary treatment is surgery, either endoscopically or via an open resection. Radiotherapy may help to improve locoregional control; however, it does not affect overall survival.[63,64] There is limited evidence suggesting that prolonged survival is realized with the addition of chemotherapy, such as dacarbazine, platinum analogues, nitrosoureas, microtubular toxins, or taxols.[65,66] Further prospective, randomized clinical trials are necessary to confirm any definitive outcome effect.

Olfactory Neuroblastoma

Olfactory neuroblastoma is an uncommon malignancy hypothesized to arise from the olfactory epithelium. Its uncertain origin has resulted in different names; however, the most common terms used in the literature are olfactory neuroblastoma and esthesioneuroblastoma. This neoplasm accounts for approximately 7% to 10% of all sinonasal malignancies, and occurs with a bimodal peak in the second and sixth decades of life.[67,68] Impairment or a loss of the sense of smell, as one might expect, is not a common presentation because the contralateral part of the olfactory system is often still preserved. The initial stage of the disease is highly correlated with survival outcome. Several clinical staging systems have evolved over the past decades: the Kadish staging system,[69] described in 1976, is the first and most commonly used staging system incorporating 3 groups: group A contains tumors confined to the nasal cavity, group B tumors involving the

paranasal sinuses, and group C tumors that extend beyond the sinonasal cavity. This system was modified by Foote and colleagues[70] with the addition of stage D, which includes cervical or distant metastasis. A third system, based on the TNM classification system, has been described by Dulguerov and Calcaterra (**Box 2**).[71] In addition, a histologic grading system reported by Hyams[72] describes 4 different grades, from Grade I (well differentiated) to Grade IV (undifferentiated). The grading is based on growth, architecture, mitotic activity, necrosis, nuclear polymorphism, rosette formation, and fibrillary stroma. There is a lack of consensus of whether this grading system is predictive of outcome. The most frequently used approach for treating olfactory neuroblastoma is a combined approach with radiotherapy given either before or after surgical resection.[73–75] Patients diagnosed with Kadish stage A or stage T1 lesions may not require adjuvant radiotherapy if clear surgical margins are achieved. To obtain adequate surgical margins, the cribriform plate is resected en bloc.[76] The classic combined anterior craniofacial resections have been replaced by expanded endoscopic approaches in selected cases, without impact on the 5-year control rate.[77–79] The 5-year disease-specific survival is reported to range from 52% to 90%.[71,75] Although olfactory neuroblastoma is not generally believed to be chemosensitive, some centers have advocated adjunctive chemotherapy to the treatment for Kadish B or C lesions. However, this combined-therapy approach has not been widely accepted.

Box 2
TNM-staging system according to Dulguerov and Calcaterra[71] for olfactory neuroblastoma

Stage	Characteristics
T1	Tumor involving nasal cavity and/or paranasal sinuses (excluding sphenoid sinus) sparing the most superior ethmoid cells
T2	Tumor involving nasal cavity and/or paranasal sinuses (including sphenoid sinus) with extension to or erosion of the cribriform plate
T3	Tumor extending into the orbit or protruding into anterior cranial fossa, without dural involvement
T4	Tumor involving the brain
N0	No cervical lymph node involvement
N1	Any form of cervical lymph node metastasis
M0	No distant metastases
M1	Any distant metastases

Sinonasal Neuroendocrine Carcinoma

Sinonasal neuroendocrine carcinoma (SNEC) is rare and accounts for fewer than 5% of malignancies of the sinonasal tract.[80] The exact histologic diagnosis of this tumor can be challenging, owing to the difficulty of differentiating SNEC from olfactory neuroblastoma, sinonasal undifferentiated carcinoma, melanoma, and other small cell tumors of the sinonasal tract. The most common sites of origin are the ethmoid sinuses and the nasal cavity, with presenting symptoms that mimic those of rhinosinusitis and other benign sinonasal disorders, frequently resulting in a delayed diagnosis.[80,81] Accordingly, involvement of the skull base (bone or orbit) negatively affects survival. In general, SNEC shows epithelial differentiation with specific histologic and immunohistochemical features, such as a high mitotic rate and positivity for keratin and synaptophysin.[82,83] SNEC is associated with a high rate of locoregional recurrence

and distant metastasis.[84,85] In a published series of 28 patients, Mitchell and colleagues[80] report a 25% recurrence of tumor in the neck and conclude that elective neck dissection should be considered in all patients considered for surgery. The ideal treatment strategy has yet to be determined. In addition to surgery and radiotherapy, systemic treatment may play a future role in the individualized management of this disease.

MANAGEMENT

In general, sinonasal malignancies do not cause symptoms until they have reached a certain size and expansion. Thus a high degree of suspicion is required to avoid delay in diagnosis. A thorough endoscopic examination with biopsy and radiographic imaging are the first steps when a suspicious lesion is present. Both computed tomography (CT) and magnetic resonance imaging (MRI) are now established as the optimum imaging assessment of

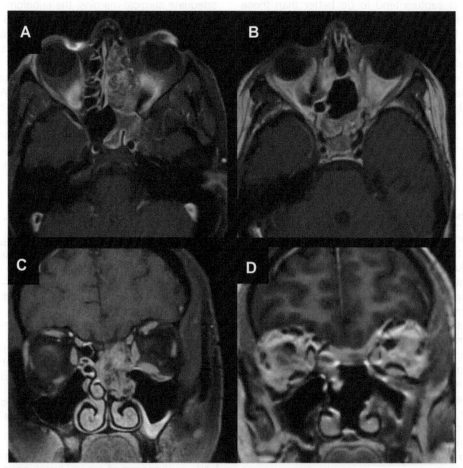

Fig. 1. (*A*) Axial and (*C*) coronal preoperative postcontrast-enhanced T1-weighted magnetic resonance images of a 40-year-old female patient with a seromucinous adenocarcinoma. Before surgery, the patient was radiated. (*B*) Axial and (*D*) coronal postoperative magnetic resonance images after an expanded endoscopic endonasal approach with nasoseptal flap showed complete removal of the tumor. All surgical margins were tumor negative.

sinonasal malignancy.[86] Haerle and colleagues[87] suggested that the radiologic evaluation in cases of sinonasal melanoma is best performed by metabolic imaging, such as ^{18}F-fluorodeoxyglucose positron emission tomography (PET), PET/CT, or PET/MRI if available. In general, metabolic imaging can be considered for initial exclusion of distant disease because the presence of such will alter the treatment plan significantly. MRI generally offers better tumor and tissue differentiation, whereas a CT scan is required to assess potential bone erosion.[88] During follow-up, MRI is considered to be the imaging modality of choice (**Fig. 1**).[89]

When exact staging is complete, a multidisciplinary oncologic discussion should take place. The optimal treatment for patients suffering from sinonasal malignancies remains to be defined, but open or endoscopic craniofacial resection followed by postoperative radiotherapy is currently considered for the vast majority of patients with locally advanced disease.

The Role of Radiotherapy

It is widely accepted that most sinonasal carcinomas are radiosensitive; however, radiosensitivity largely depends on the histology and growth rate of the tumor.[6] In the case of localized disease, radiation, either as a single-modality treatment or with combination treatment, offers a limited survival advantage.[1] Blanch and colleagues[8] reported no survival benefit with the addition of radiotherapy to surgery for early-stage disease Therefore, the primary treatment of choice for most sinonasal carcinomas is complete surgical tumor resection with adjuvant radiotherapy with or without systemic therapy.[6,90] There have been some published reports regarding intraoperative high-dose brachytherapy.[91] However, these studies are limited by small sample sizes and concern only patients with locally advanced or recurrent disease.

The Role of Chemotherapy

There are some preliminary reports on concurrent chemoradiation in sinonasal carcinomas, albeit limited to advanced SCC and SNUC.[92,93] Other literature describes the use of systemic treatments for specific histology subtypes of sinonasal carcinomas dependent on location and number of metastases. There is a role described in the literature for local chemotherapy using 5-fluorouracil in the treatment of adenocarcinoma, or as an adjuvant after minimal invasive surgical clearance.[94,95]

In the future, substantial improvements in prognosis will likely depend on the development and utilization of histology-specific and personally-directed systemic treatments.

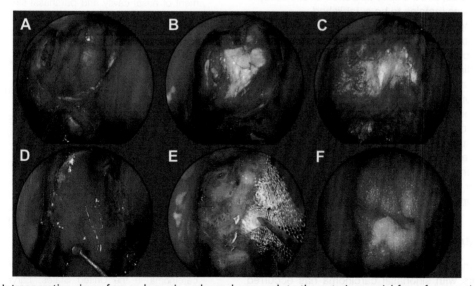

Fig. 2. Intraoperative view of an endoscopic endonasal approach to the anterior cranial fossa for resection and reconstruction of the 40-year-old woman in **Fig. 1** with a seromucinous adenocarcinoma. (*A*) View of the anterior cranial base after resection of the tumor, septum, cribriform plate, and dura. Olfactory bulb on the left side was resected. (*B*) Fascia lata was harvested and was put between the brain and dural edges. As second layer (*C*), artificial dura substitute was layered above the fascia lata graft and dural edges. The vascularized nasoseptal flap (*D*) was placed as a third layer over the artificial dura. The graft was further overlaid with Surgicel (*E*) and sealed with fibrin glue. Loose pieces of Gelfoam were placed over the reconstruction site. At the end of the procedure (*F*), a 24F Foley catheter balloon was placed and inflated to keep the grafts in place.

The Role of Surgery

There is a general consensus that the outcome of any alternative method of treatment should be compared with anterior craniofacial resection.[96,97] A surgical paradigm shift was initiated in the late 1990s with the introduction of endoscopic surgery as an exclusive approach or in combination with a frontal craniotomy.[98–100] Since then, endoscopic procedures have been compared with open approaches with regard to oncologic safety, outcome, and morbidity. According to Nicolai and colleagues,[77] the difficulty of exposing tumor margins does not impede a complete endoscopic resection. Only smaller lesions may be resected en bloc, whereas larger lesions are resected in a stepwise technique without compromising the oncologic safety. Hanna and colleagues[101] concluded that with appropriate use of adjuvant therapy, endoscopic resection of sinonasal cancer results in acceptable oncologic outcomes. For successful outcomes, endoscopic resection warrants the correct selection of cases, and should be performed by surgeons with experience in endoscopic techniques and oncologic principles. In an international collaborative study, there was an overall mortality rate of 4.7% and an overall postoperative complication rate of 36.3% using an open approach.[102] Quality-of-life measures were mainly addressed for open, craniofacial procedures, and the specific benefit of endoscopic techniques remains to be established.

An important goal of reconstruction in both open and endoscopic procedures is the separation of the sinonasal tract from cranial cavity to prevent ascending infections, cerebrospinal fluid (CSF) leaks, and pneumocephalus (**Fig. 2**). Different types of potential closures have been described, and innovative procedures such as vascularized pedicled or free flaps after an endoscopic or open approach, respectively, have reduced the postoperative complication rate. In the authors' experience, the use of vascularized free tissue transfer has substantially reduced the incidence of meningitis, CSF leaks, and pneumocephalus.[103]

SUMMARY

Over the last 40 years, improved prognosis in patients with sinonasal carcinoma has occurred as a result of advances in techniques of both evaluation and treatment. Despite these improvements, sinonasal carcinomas remain a challenging disease with high morbidity, low regional and distant disease control, and poor survival. However, future advancements to improve patient outcomes and survival include early detection, identification of tumor biological markers, and surgical innovations to provide superior access and minimize morbidity.

REFERENCES

1. Turner JH, Reh DD. Incidence and survival in patients with sinonasal cancer: a historical analysis of population-based data. Head Neck 2012;34(6): 877–85.
2. Lund VJ, Stammberger H, Nicolai P, et al. European position paper on endoscopic management of tumours of the nose, paranasal sinuses and skull base. Rhinol Suppl 2010;1:1–143.
3. Myers LL, Nussenbaum B, Bradford CR, et al. Paranasal sinus malignancies: an 18-year single institution experience. Laryngoscope 2002;112: 1964–9.
4. Waldron J, Witterick I. Paranasal sinus cancer: caveats and controversies. World J Surg 2003;27: 849–55.
5. Khademi B, Moradi A, Hoseini S, et al. Malignant neoplasms of the sinonasal tract: report of 71 patients and literature review and analysis. Oral Maxillofac Surg 2009;13:191–9.
6. Dulguerov P, Jacobsen MS, Allal AS, et al. Nasal and paranasal sinus carcinoma: are we making progress? A series of 220 patients and a systematic review. Cancer 2001;92:3012–29.
7. Hoppe BS, Stegman LD, Zelefsky MJ, et al. Treatment of nasal cavity and paranasal sinus cancer with modern radiotherapy techniques in the postoperative setting: the MSKCC experience. Int J Radiat Oncol Biol Phys 2007;67:691–702.
8. Blanch JL, Ruiz AM, Alos L, et al. Treatment of 125 sinonasal tumors: prognostic factors, outcome, and follow-up. Otolaryngol Head Neck Surg 2004; 131:973–6.
9. Grau C, Jakobsen MH, Harbo G, et al. Sino-nasal cancer in Denmark 1982-1991: a nationwide survey. Acta Oncol 2001;40:19–23.
10. Osguthorpe JD, Richardson M. Frontal sinus malignancies. Otolaryngol Clin North Am 2001;34: 269–81.
11. DeMonte F, Ginsberg LE, Clayman GL. Primary malignant tumors of the sphenoid sinus. Neurosurgery 2000;46:1084–91.
12. Sikora AG, Toniolo P, DeLacure MD. The changing demographics of head and neck squamous cell carcinoma in the United States. Laryngoscope 2004;114:1915–23.
13. Lund VJ. Malignancy of the nose and sinuses: epidemiological and aetiological considerations. Rhinology 1991;29:57–68.
14. Roush GC. Epidemiology of cancer of the nose and paranasal sinuses, current concepts. Head Neck Surg 1979;2:3–11.

15. Luce D, Leclerc A, Begin D, et al. Sinonasal cancer and occupational exposures: a pooled data analysis of 12 case-control studies. Cancer Causes Control 2002;13:147–57.

16. McKay SP, Gregoire L, Lonardo F, et al. Human papillomavirus (HPV) transcripts in malignant inverted papilloma are from integrated HPV DNA. Laryngoscope 2005;115:1428–31.

17. Syrjaenen KJ. HPV infections in benign and malignant sinonasal lesions. J Clin Pathol 2003; 56:174–81.

18. Alos L, Moyano S, Nadal A, et al. Human papillomaviruses are identified in a subgroup of sinonasal squamous cell carcinomas with favorable outcome. Cancer 2009;115:2701–9.

19. Ohngren LG. Malignant tumours of the maxilloethmoidal region. Acta Otolaryngol 1993;19:101–6.

20. Edge SB, Byrd DR, Compton CC, et al, editors. AJCC cancer staging manual. 7th edition. New York: Springer; 2010.

21. Patel SG, Singh B, Polluri A, et al. Craniofacial surgery for malignant skull base surgery. Cancer 2003;98:1170–87.

22. Harvey RJ, Gallagher RM, Sacks R. Extended endoscopic techniques for sinonasal resections. Otolaryngol Clin North Am 2010;43:6113–638.

23. Barnes L, Everson JW, Reichart P, et al. Pathology and genetics of head and neck tumors. Lyon (France): IARC Press; 2005.

24. Wenig BM. Undifferentiated malignant neoplasms of the sinonasal tract. Arch Pathol Lab Med 2009; 133:699–712.

25. Woodson GE, Robbins T, Michaels L. Inverted papilloma. Consideration in treatment. Arch Otolaryngol 1985;11:806–11.

26. Tanvetyanon T, Qin D, Padhya T, et al. Survival outcomes of squamous cell carcinoma arising from sinonasal inverted papilloma: report of 6 cases with systematic review and pooled analysis. Am J Otolaryngol 2009;30:38–43.

27. Tufano RP, Mokadam NA, Montone KT, et al. Malignant tumors of the nose and paranasal sinuses: hospital of the University of Pennsylvania experience 1990-1997. Am J Rhinol 1999;13:117–23.

28. Wienecke JA, Thompson LD, Wenig BM. Basaloid squamous cell carcinoma of the sinonasal tract. Cancer 1999;85:841–54.

29. Hayashi T, Nonaka S, Bandoh N, et al. Treatment outcome of maxillary sinus squamous cell carcinoma. Cancer 2001;92:1495–503.

30. Tiwari R, Hardillo JA, Mehta D, et al. Squamous cell carcinoma of maxillary sinus. Head Neck 2000;22: 164–9.

31. Kim GE, Chung EJ, Lim JJ, et al. Clinical significance of neck node metastasis in squamous cell carcinoma of the maxillary antrum. Am J Otolaryngol 1999;20:383–90.

32. Kida A, Endo S, Iida H, et al. Clinical assessment of squamous cell carcinoma of the nasal cavity proper. Auris Nasus Larynx 1995;22:172–7.

33. Kleinsasser O, Schroeder HG. Adenocarcinomas of the inner nose after exposure to wood dust. Morphological findings and relationships between histopathology and clinical behaviour in 79 cases. Arch Otorhinolaryngol 1988;245:1–5.

34. Barnes L. Intestinal-type adenocarcinoma of the nasal cavity and the paranasal sinuses. Am J Surg Pathol 1986;10:192–202.

35. Gnepp DR, Heffner DK. Mucosal origin of sinonasal tract adenomatous neoplasms. Mod Pathol 1989;2: 365–71.

36. Stoll D, Bebar JB, Truilhe Y, et al. Ethmoid adenocarcinomas: retrospective study of 76 patients. Rev Laryngol Otol Rhinol 2002;122:21–9.

37. Knegt PP, Ah-See KW, van de Velden LA, et al. Adenocarcinoma of the ethmoid sinus complex: surgical debulking and topical fluorouracil may be the optimal treatment. Arch Otolaryngol Head Neck Surg 2001;127:141–6.

38. Perzin KH, Gullane P, Clairmont AC. Adenoid cystic carcinomas arising in salivary glands: a correlation of histologic features and clinical course. Cancer 1978;42:265–82.

39. Khan AJ, DiGiovanna MP, Ross DA, et al. Adenoid cystic carcinoma: a retrospective clinical review. Int J Cancer 2001;96:149–58.

40. Spiro RH, Huvos AG, Strong EW. Adenoid cystic carcinoma of salivary origin: a clinicopathologic study of 242 cases. Am J Surg 1974;128: 512–20.

41. Kim GE, Park HC, Keum KC, et al. Adenoid cystic carcinoma of the maxillary antrum. Am J Otolaryngol 1999;20:77–84.

42. Jones AS, Hamilton JW, Rowley H, et al. Adenoid cystic carcinoma of the head and neck. Clin Otolaryngol Allied Sci 1997;22:434–43.

43. Spiro RH. Distant metastasis in adenoid cystic carcinoma of salivary origin. Am J Surg 1997;174: 495–8.

44. Naficy S, Disher MJ, Esclamado RM. Adenoid cystic carcinoma of the paranasal sinuses. Am J Rhinol 1999;13:311–4.

45. Pitman KT, Prokopakis EP, Aydogan B, et al. The role of skull base surgery for the treatment of adenoid cystic carcinoma of the sinonasal tract. Head Neck 1999;21:402–7.

46. Airoldi M, Pedani F, Succo G, et al. Phase II randomized trial comparing vinorelbine versus vinorelbine plus cisplatin in patients with recurrent salivary gland malignancies. Cancer 2001;91: 541–7.

47. Wolfish EB, Nelson BL, Thompson LDR. Sinonasal tract mucoepidermoid carcinoma: a clinicopathologic and immunophenotypic study of 19 cases

combined with a comprehensive review of the literature. Head Neck Pathol 2012;6(2):191–207.

48. Loh KS, Barker E, Bruch G, et al. Prognostic factors in malignancy of the minor salivary glands. Head Neck 2009;31:58–63.

49. Neto AG, Pineda-Daboin K, Spencer ML, et al. Sinonasal acinic cell carcinoma: a clinicopathologic study of four cases. Head Neck 2005;27:603–7.

50. Luna MA. Sialoblastoma and epithelial tumors in children, their morphologic spectrum and distribution by age. Adv Anat Pathol 1999;6:287–92.

51. Laskawi R, Rodel R, Zirk A, et al. Retrospective analysis of 35 patients with acinic cell carcinoma of the parotid gland. J Oral Maxillofac Surg 1998; 56:440–3.

52. Frierson HF Jr, Mills SE, Fechner RE, et al. Sinonasal undifferentiated carcinoma: an aggressive neoplasm derived from schneiderian epithelium and distinct from olfactory neuroblastoma. Am J Surg Pathol 1986;10:771–9.

53. Tanzler ED, Morris CG, Orlando CA, et al. Management of sinonasal undifferentiated carcinoma. Head Neck 2008;30:595–9.

54. Gorelick J, Ross D, Marentette L, et al. Sinonasal undifferentiated carcinoma: case series and review of the literature. Neurosurgery 2000;47:750–4.

55. Cerilli LA, Holst VA, Brandwein MS, et al. Sinonasal undifferentiated carcinoma: immunohistochemical profile and lack of EBV association. Am J Surg Pathol 2001;25:156–63.

56. Deutsch BD, Levine PA, Stewart FM, et al. Sinonasal undifferentiated carcinoma: a ray of hope. Otolaryngol Head Neck Surg 1993;108:697–700.

57. Reiersen DA, Pahilan ME, Devaiah AK. Meta-analysis of treatment outcomes for sinonasal undifferentiated carcinoma. Otolaryngol Head Neck Surg 2012;147(1):7–14.

58. Ganly I, Patel SG, Singh B, et al. Craniofacial resection for malignant melanoma of the skull base. Arch Otolaryngol Head Neck Surg 2006; 132:73–8.

59. Batsakis JG, Suarez P, El-Naggar AK. Mucosal melanomas of the head and neck. Ann Otol Rhinol Laryngol 1998;107:626–30.

60. Regauer S, Anderhuber W, Richtig E, et al. Primary mucosal melanomas of the nasal cavity and paranasal sinuses. A clinicopathological analysis of 14 cases. APMIS 1998;106:403–10.

61. Lund VJ, Howard DJ, Harding L, et al. Management options and survival in malignant melanoma of the sinonasal mucosa. Laryngoscope 1999; 109:208–11.

62. Dauer EH, Lewis JE, Rohlinger AL, et al. Sinonasal melanoma: a clinicopathologic review of 61 cases. Otolaryngol Head Neck Surg 2008;138:347–52.

63. Lund VJ, Chisholm EJ, Howard DJ, et al. Sinonasal malignant melanoma: an analysis of 115 cases assessing outcomes of surgery, postoperative radiotherapy and endoscopic resection. Rhinology 2012;50:203–10.

64. Thomson LD, Wieneke JA, Miettinen M. Sinonasal tract and nasopharyngeal melanomas: a clinicopathologic study of 115 cases with a proposed staging system. Am J Surg Pathol 2003;27: 594–611.

65. Lengyel E, Glide K, Remenar E, et al. Malignant mucosal melanoma of the head and neck. Pathol Oncol Res 2003;9:7–12.

66. Wang J, Murakami T, Hakamata Y, et al. Gene gun-mediated oral mucosal transfer of interleukin 12 cDNA coupled with an irradiated melanoma vaccine in a hamster model: successful treatment of oral melanoma and distant skin lesion. Cancer Gene Ther 2001;8:705–12.

67. Morita A, Ebersold MJ, Olsen KD, et al. Esthesioneuroblastoma: prognosis and management. Neurosurgery 1993;32:706–15.

68. Spiro JD, Soo KC, Spiro RH. Nonsquamous cell malignant neoplasms of the nasal cavities and paranasal sinuses. Head Neck 1995;17:114–8.

69. Kadish S, Goodman M, Wang CC. Olfactory neuroblastoma. A clinical analysis of 17 cases. Cancer 1976;37:1571–6.

70. Foote RL, Morita A, Ebersold MJ, et al. Esthesioneuroblastoma: the role of radiation therapy. Int J Radiat Oncol Biol Phys 1993;27:835–42.

71. Dulguerov P, Calcaterra T. Esthesioneuroblastoma: the UCLA experience 1970-1990. Laryngoscope 1992;102:843–9.

72. Hyams VJ. Olfactory neuroblastoma. In: Hyams V, Batsakis Michaels L, editors. Tumours of the upper respiratory tract and ear. Washington, DC: Armed Forces Institute of Pathology; 1998. p. 240–8.

73. Dulguerov P, Allal AS, Calcaterra TC. Esthesioneuroblastoma: a meta- analysis and review. Lancet Oncol 2001;2:683–90.

74. Rastogi M, Bhatt M, Chufal K, et al. Esthesioneuroblastoma treated with non-craniofacial resection surgery followed by combined chemotherapy and radiotherapy: an alternative approach in limited resources. Jpn J Clin Oncol 2006;36:613–9.

75. Bachar G, Goldstein DP, Shah M, et al. Esthesioneuroblastoma: the Princess Margaret Hospital experience. Head Neck 2008;30:1607–14.

76. Girod D, Hanna E, Marentette L. Esthesioneuroblastoma. Head Neck 2001;23:500–5.

77. Nicolai P, Battaglia P, Bignami M, et al. Endoscopic surgery for malignant tumors of the sinonasal tract and adjacent skull base: a 10-year experience. Am J Rhinol 2008;22:308–16.

78. Folbe A, Herzallah I, Duvvuri U, et al. Endoscopic endonasal resection of esthesioneuroblastoma: a multicenter study. Am J Rhinol Allergy 2009;23: 91–4.

79. Villaret AB, Yakirevitch A, Bizzoni A, et al. Endoscopic transnasal craniectomy in the management of selected sinonasal malignancies. Am J Rhinol Allergy 2010;24:60–5.

80. Mitchell EH, Diaz A, Yilmaz T, et al. Multimodality treatment for sinonasal neuroendocrine carcinoma. Head Neck 2011. [Epub ahead of print].

81. Smith SR, Som P, Fahmy A, et al. A clinicopathological study of sinonasal neuroendocrine carcinoma and sinonasal undifferentiated carcinoma. Laryngoscope 2000;110:1617–22.

82. Cordes B, Williams MD, Tirado Y, et al. Molecular and phenotypic analysis of poorly differentiated sinonasal neoplasms: an integrated approach for early diagnosis and classification. Hum Pathol 2009;40:283–92.

83. Iezzoni JC, Mills SE. "Undifferentiated" small round cell tumors of the sinonasal tract. Differential diagnosis update. Am J Clin Pathol 2005;124: 110–21.

84. Rosenthal DI, Barker JL Jr, El-Naggar AK, et al. Sinonasal malignancies with neuroendocrine differentiation: patterns of failure according to histologic phenotype. Cancer 2004;101:2567–73.

85. Perez-Ordonez B, Caruana SM, Huvos AG, et al. Small cell neuroendocrine carcinoma of the nasal cavity and paranasal sinuses. Hum Pathol 1998; 29:826–32.

86. Lloyd G, Lund VJ, Howard D, et al. Optimum imaging for sinonasal malignancy. J Laryngol Otol 2000;114:557–62.

87. Haerle SK, Soyka MB, Fischer DR, et al. The value of ^{18}F-FDG-PET/CT imaging for sinonasal malignant melanoma. Eur Arch Otorhinolaryngol 2012; 269:127–33.

88. Lund VJ, Howard DJ, Lloyd GA. CT evaluation of paranasal sinus tumours for cranio-facial resection. Br J Radiol 1989;11:439–46.

89. Lund VJ, Howard DJ, Lloyd GA, et al. Magnetic resonance imaging of paranasal sinus tumours for craniofacial resection. Head Neck 1989;11: 279–83.

90. Jansen EP, Keus RB, Hilgers FJ, et al. Does the combination of radiotherapy and debulking surgery favor survival in paranasal carcinoma? Int J Radiat Oncol Biol Phys 2000;48:27–35.

91. Nag S, Tippin D, Grecula J, et al. Intraoperative high-dose-rate brachytherapy for paranasal sinus tumors. Int J Radiat Oncol Biol Phys 2004;58: 155–60.

92. Nishimura G, Tsukuda M, Mikami Y, et al. The efficacy and safety of concurrent chemoradiotherapy for maxillary sinus squamous cell carcinoma. Auris, Nasus, Larynx 2009;36:547–54.

93. Enepekides DJ. Sinonasal undifferentiated carcinoma: an update. Curr Opin Otolaryngol Head Neck Surg 2005;13:222–5.

94. Sato Y, Morita M, Takahashi HO, et al. Combined surgery, radiotherapy, and regional chemotherapy in carcinoma of the paranasal sinuses. Cancer 1970;25:571–9.

95. Knegt PP, deJong PC, van Ander JG, et al. Carcinoma of the paranasal sinuses. Results of a prospective pilot study. Cancer 1985;56:57–62.

96. Lund VJ, Howard DJ, Wei W. Endoscopic resection of malignant tumors of the nose and sinuses. Am J Rhinol 2007;21:89–94.

97. Batra PS, Citardi MJ, Worley S, et al. Resection of anterior skull base tumors: comparison of combined traditional endoscopic techniques. Am J Rhinol 2005;19:521–8.

98. Stammberger H, Anderhuber W, Wlach C, et al. Possibilities and limitations of endoscopic management of nasal and paranasal sinus malignancies. Acta Otorhinolaryngol Belg 1999;53:199–205.

99. Yuen AP, Fung CF, Hung KN. Endoscopic crranionasal resection of anterior skull base tumor. Am J Otolaryngol 1997;118:431–3.

100. Thaler ER, Kotapka M, Lanza DC, et al. Endoscopically assisted anterior cranial skull base resection of sinonasal tumors. Am J Rhinol 1999;13:303–10.

101. Hanna E, DeMonte F, Ibrahim S, et al. Endoscopic resection of sinonasal cancers with and without craniotomy: oncologic results. Arch Otolaryngol Head Neck Surg 2009;1135:1219–24.

102. Ganly I, Patel SG, Singh B. Complications of craniofacial resection for malignant tumors of the skull base: report of an International Collaborative Study. Head Neck 2005;27:445–51.

103. Neligan P, Mulholland S, Gullane P. Flap selection in cranial base surgery. Plast Reconstr Surg 1996;98:1159–66.

Esthesioneuroblastoma

Thomas J. Ow, MD, MS[a], Diana Bell, MD[b],
Michael E. Kupferman, MD[a],
Franco DeMonte, MD, FRCSC[a,c,d], Ehab Y. Hanna, MD[a,c],*

KEYWORDS

- Esthesioneuroblastoma • Multimodality treatment • Endoscopic resection

KEY POINTS

- Esthesioneuroblastoma is a rare malignancy that arises in the midline of the anterior skull base.
- Accurate pathologic diagnosis relies on immunohistochemical evaluation in poorly differentiated cases, and discrimination from other neuroendocrine tumors is crucial for appropriate treatment and prognostication.
- Several staging systems exist, but none have been universally adopted.
- Lymph node metastatic disease increases the likelihood of recurrence and portends a poor prognosis.
- Multimodality treatment is commonly used. Complete surgical resection via anterior craniofacial resection with postoperative irradiation has been the most commonly advocated regimen for resectable disease. Endoscopic-assisted or complete endoscopic resection techniques are increasingly being used.

INTRODUCTION

Esthesioneuroblastoma (ENB) was first described by Berger and Richard in 1924.[1] It has been characterized as a rare malignant neoplasm of the sinonasal cavity that arises in the superior portion of the nasal vault. Since its first description, ENB has been referenced under several names, but the accepted terms at this time are "esthesioneuroblastoma" and "olfactory neuroblastoma." The exact origin of this tumor, both the location and cell type, is under debate. Proposed anatomic sites of origin include Jacobson organ, the sphenopalatine ganglion, the ectodermal olfactory placode, Loci's ganglion, sympathetic ganglia of the nasal mucosa, and the nasal mucosa itself.[2,3] However, the most likely site of origin, and the one most generally accepted, is the basal neural cells of the olfactory mucosa.[2–4] The olfactory epithelium is unique in the human nervous system in that it is capable of regeneration and the histologic organization of the olfactory organ reflects this ability. Several cell types are present: the mature olfactory neuroepithelial cells, a basal layer of stem cells that repopulate the differentiated epithelium, sustentacular supporting cells, and flat cells forming the ducts of Bowman in the olfactory lamina propria.[5] ENB seems to be of neuronal or neural crest origin, this idea is supported by the neural filaments present in tumor cells.[6] Also, molecular analysis suggests that ENB is derived from immature olfactory neurons.[4]

Disclosures: None.
[a] Department of Head and Neck Surgery, The University of Texas MD Anderson Cancer Center, 1515 Holcombe Boulevard, Houston, TX 77030, USA; [b] Department of Pathology, The University of Texas MD Anderson Cancer Center, 1515 Holcombe Boulevard, Houston, TX 77030, USA; [c] Department of Neurosurgery, The University of Texas MD Anderson Cancer Center, 1515 Holcombe Boulevard, Houston, TX 77030, USA; [d] Department of Neurosurgery, Baylor College of Medicine, The University of Texas MD Anderson Cancer Center, 1515 Holcombe Boulevard, Houston, TX 77030, USA
* Corresponding author.
E-mail address: EYHanna@mdanderson.org

Neurosurg Clin N Am 24 (2013) 51–65
http://dx.doi.org/10.1016/j.nec.2012.08.005

Regardless of its origin, several factors have presented challenges to the characterization and treatment of ENB. First, the tumor is very rare, making it a difficult entity to study. Second, ENB can be difficult to differentiate from several other neoplasms. Third, ENB itself can demonstrate a wide spectrum of clinical behavior, ranging from relatively indolent to both locally aggressive and metastatic. Despite these challenges, the diagnosis and management of ENB has progressed significantly during the last 30 years.

EPIDEMIOLOGY

Malignancies of the sinonasal tract are rare, and ENB is uncommon even among neoplasms that fall within this category, accounting for roughly 3% of all tumors found in the nasal cavity.[2] No apparent causal factors have been identified for this disease. There is, perhaps, a very slight male predominance reported among large series, with an approximate 55% male to 45% female distribution[2,7–9] (Ow TJ, Hanna EY, Roberts DB, et al. Multimodality therapy optimizes long-term outcome in patients with esthesioneuroblastoma. Unpublished data, manuscript under review, 2012). ENB has been reported across several ethnicities, but published cases have been largely among the white population[9] (Ow TJ, Hanna EY, Roberts DB, et al. Multimodality therapy optimizes long-term outcome in patients with esthesioneuroblastoma. Unpublished data, manuscript under review, 2012). Although some investigators have suggested that the age at which ENB develops has a bimodal distribution,[10] this is not supported by recent large reviews, which more accurately suggest that the disease has been diagnosed across all decades, with a peak in the fifth or sixth decade.[2,7,9]

ANATOMY OF THE ANTERIOR SKULL BASE

The following is a brief description of the region of the anterior skull base. For more detail, the reader is referred to the work by Rhoton[11] and the article by Pinheiro-Neto and colleagues.[12] The anterior skull base can be divided into the medial and lateral compartments. The medial compartment is made up of the ethmoid, sphenoid, and frontal bones. The anterior-most aspect of the bony skull base is composed of the frontal bones, housing the pyramidal frontal sinuses. Inferiorly, the nasal cavity is found anteriorly and the sphenoid body housing the sphenoid sinus is found posteriorly. On the endocranial side, the crista galli is found at the midline. The gyri rectus, the anterior cerebral arteries, and the olfactory bulbs rest on the anteromedial base of the skull. Here, the roof of the ethmoid bone forms the cribriform plate anteriorly, where the olfactory rootlets pierce the bony skull base to enter the nasal cavity, and where an emissary vein traverses the foramen caecum. It is from this region the ENB is thought to arise. Posteriorly, the planum sphenoidale is found with the sella turcica housing the pituitary gland. Within the nasal cavity, the perpendicular plate of the ethmoid joins the vomer at the midline to make up the posterior nasal septum. The lateral plates of the ethmoid contribute to the medial orbital walls. The superior turbinates project from the roof of the ethmoid into the nasal cavity, lateral to the cribriform plate. The sphenoethmoid recesses and ostia to the sphenoid sinus can be found superior and posterior to the superior turbinates.

The lateral portion of the anterior skull base is the region of the orbit. Endocranially, the orbital gyri and middle cerebral arteries rest on the anterolateral skull base. The roof of the orbit is formed from the lesser wing of the sphenoid bone and the zygomatic bone. The inferior bony orbit is formed from the zygomatic, maxillary, and palatine bones. The medial wall of the orbit is formed from the maxilla, lacrimal bone, and ethmoid bones. There are several important foramina in the lateral portion of the anterior skull base. The anterior and posterior ethmoidal foramina are conduits for the branches of the ophthalmic artery bearing the same names, found traversing the superomedial orbital walls from the orbit to the superior nasal cavity. The supratrochlear foramen medially and the supraorbital foramen laterally house the neurovascular bundles superior to the orbits that supply the soft tissues of the forehead. In the posterior orbit, the optic canal is formed by the frontal bone and the lesser wing of the sphenoid, and the optic nerve and ophthalmic arteries are transmitted from intracranial to the orbit through this structure. The superior orbital fissure is found between the lesser wing and greater wing of the sphenoid. The oculomotor nerve (CN III), trochlear nerve (CN IV), lacrimal, frontal, nasociliary branches of the ophthalmic (CN V3) nerve, abducens nerve (CN VI), the ophthalmic vein, and sympathetic fibers from the cavernous sinus all pass through the superior orbital fissure. The inferior orbital fissure is found between the greater wing of the sphenoid and the anterior orbital floor formed by the maxillary and palatine bones. The maxillary nerve and its zygomatic branch, as well as the ascending branches from the pterygopalatine ganglion, can be found traversing the inferior orbital fissure. The adjacent infraorbital canal transmits the infraorbital artery and vein, which exit the infraorbital foramen to the soft tissues of the cheek.

Access to the anterior cranial base can be achieved via a bifrontal craniotomy, a subfrontal-transglabellar approach, a transnasal approach, and a transmaxillary-transnasal route. A detailed understanding of the anatomy of the midface, nasal cavity, paranasal sinuses, orbit, and anterior cranial fossa are crucial to successful surgery for ENB.

CLINICAL PRESENTATION

ENB, like all sinonasal tumors, can grow insidiously, and the common symptoms are very nonspecific and commonly associated with benign processes. A usual delay of 6 to 12 months between the onset of symptoms and diagnosis of ENB has been reported.[13,14] Symptomatology is related to the anatomic structures affected by mass effect or local invasion. The most common presenting symptoms are nasal obstruction, followed by epistaxis.[2,3,8,10,13–15] Other nasal symptoms include headache, facial pain, "sinusitis," hyposmia or anosmia, or an asymptomatic nasal mass.[2,8,10,14] Visual symptoms occur when the orbit is invaded and include diplopia, vision loss, proptosis, and epiphora.[2,8,10,15] Intracranial invasion can rarely produce additional symptoms, including effects secondary to pituitary dysfunction, such as diabetes insipidus or hormonal disturbance, blindness secondary to effects on the optic nerves and chiasm, or neurologic symptoms secondary to mass effect or intracranial hypertension.[2,15] Because symptoms associated with ENB are nonspecific and mimic those of benign sinonasal processes, an increased index of suspicion is crucial to improve early detection of these tumors. It has been suggested that unilateral symptoms and recurrent epistaxis for more than 1 to 2 months warrant more thorough investigation for a possible malignant process.[3] It has been shown that patients with ENB present with unilateral symptoms more often than bilateral symptoms.[8] One study has also compared patients diagnosed preoperatively with bilateral polyposis to those with unilateral polyps and found that neoplastic and malignant processes were exclusively diagnosed in the group with unilateral findings.[16]

DIAGNOSTIC WORKUP

Any patient with a history that is suspicious for a sinonasal tumor deserves a thorough neurologic, ophthalmologic, and head and neck examination. Cranial nerve abnormalities, including deficits in olfaction, facial paresthesias, ophthalmoplegia, and visual field deficits are concerning and should be noted. Middle ear effusion may be identified if the eustachian tube is obstructed. Proptosis and conjunctival injection are, of course, significant findings for orbital involvement. Nasal endoscopy is a necessity. Flexible fiberoptic endoscopy has the advantages of greater patient comfort, more facile assessment of the entirety of the nasal cavity, and the ability to concurrently evaluate the pharynx and larynx, whereas rigid nasal endoscopy offers the advantage of improved resolution and the ability to manipulate with a second instrument such as a suction or forceps.

After a mass is identified, imaging is needed for qualitative evaluation and staging. High-resolution sinus CT scan with intravenous contrast should be performed[3,10] and the protocol should request thin (3 mm) sections through the skull base and paranasal sinuses. ENB metastasizes to the neck in 20% to 25% of cases, though only approximately 5% to 8% of patients present with cervical metastases.[17] Therefore, a CT scan of the neck should be included in the diagnostic workup, as well, to evaluate for regional metastasis. Views in three dimensions—axial, coronal, and sagittal—are optimal, and a protocol amenable to image-guidance is useful if there is a consideration for endoscopic management. MRI is complementary[3,10] and both imaging modalities are recommended. ENB is most typically hypointense compared with brain gray matter on T1-weighted MRI and should enhance with gadolinium. T2-weighted images show an isointense or hyperintense mass. Whereas CT scan is the optimal modality for evaluation of bony involvement (particularly the lamina papyracea, cribriform plate, and fovea ethmoidalis), MRI provides better discrimination between tumor and secretions and optimal evaluation of orbital and intracranial or brain parenchymal involvement.

After adequate examination on physical examination and imaging, biopsy is the next important step in securing a diagnosis. The authors generally recommend intraoperative biopsy under general anesthesia for any sinonasal mass, particularly lesions suspicious for malignancy, those deep in the nasal cavity, and those near the skull base or orbit. Biopsy is ideally performed after imaging has been reviewed to determine the vascularity of the mass. Bleeding from a vascular tumor is best managed in the operative setting. Because ENB can often be easily confused with several other sinonasal malignancies without careful immunohistologic characterization (see later discussion) it is best to reserve definitive management after thorough pathologic review on permanent section.

HISTOLOGIC FEATURES

When the tumor is well-differentiated, ENB forms submucosal, sharply-demarcated nests or sheets of cells, often separated by richly vascular or hyalinized fibrous stroma. The cells are often uniform, with sparse cytoplasm and round or ovoid nuclei with punctuate ("salt-and-pepper") chromatin and nucleoli that are either small or absent. The mitotic rate can be variable, but is usually low. ENB is characterized by fibrillary cytoplasm and interdigitating neuronal processes (neuropil). The cells can be arranged in glandular rings with a true lumen (called Flexner-Wintersteiner rosette) or pseudorosette (Homer-Wright pseudorosette). Examples of these characteristic features[3,18,19] are presented in **Figs. 1** and **2**.

ENB can be more difficult to diagnose when the tumor is less differentiated, with increasing pleomorphism, higher mitotic rate, and areas of necrosis (see later discussion of Hyams' grading), which can make this entity difficult to distinguish from other sinonasal tumors, particularly small blue cell tumors (see later discussion of sinonasal tumors considered in the differential diagnosis). In difficult cases, a panel of immunohistochemical markers is crucial to the establishment of a definitive diagnosis. ENB typically shows diffuse staining with neuron-specific enolase, synaptophysin, and chromogranin. Cytokeratins, glial fibrillary acid protein, neurofibrillary protein, β-tubulin, microtubule-associated protein, vimentin, epithelial membrane antigen, Leu-7 (CD57), and CD56 can all show variable reactivity. Desmin and myogenin, vimentin, and actin are negative, an important marker ruling out rhabdomyosarcoma. S-100 is variably positive, but positive cells are usually limited to the periphery of neoplastic nests, corresponding to sustentacular cells. This characteristic pattern differentiates ENB from sinonasal melanoma. FLI1 is negative, as is the EWS/FLI1 chimeric transcript, ruling out the rare diagnosis of peripheral neuroectodermal tumor or Ewing sarcoma. The typical immunohistochemistry panel and expected findings in ENB and other sinonasal tumors in the differential diagnosis are summarized in **Table 1**.[3,18,19] Typical staining patterns are exemplified in **Fig. 3**.

Electron microscopy, though less commonly used, can be helpful in the diagnosis of ENB. Typical findings are tumor cells with cytoplasmic dense-core neurosecretory granules, and neurite-like cell processes containing neurofilaments or neurotubules.[18,19]

GRADING SYSTEM

One grading system exists for ENB, which was described by Hyams in 1988.[20] This system scores mitotic activity, nuclear polymorphism, amount of fibrillary matrix, rosette formation, and amount of necrosis seen. Categories are scored, and characteristics are organized into four tiers (**Table 2**). When this system has been reviewed in the literature to compare grade to survival, grades I and II, and grades III and IV are often combined.[3] Data supporting the value of this system for prognostication have been mixed. A report by Zafereo and colleagues[14] did not find that Hyams' grade was associated with disease-specific or recurrence-free survival. In Dulguerov and colleagues[3] meta-analysis, only five studies were identified that evaluated Hyams' grading, and collectively grade III and IV tumors were associated with decreased survival. Some flaws of the Hyams' grading scale are that is subjective, leading to variable grading between pathologists, and there is sampling error when the entire tumor is not examined, as in

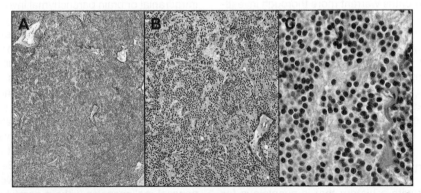

Fig. 1. Characteristic histologic features of lower grade ENB. (*A, B*) low-power (2×, 10×) magnification demonstrates monotonous cells growing in sharply demarcated nests and sheets. (*C*) High-power (40×) view demonstrates cells with round nuclei and punctuates "salt-and-pepper" chromatin embedded in a neurofibrillary stroma. See Hyams' grading system (see **Table 2**).

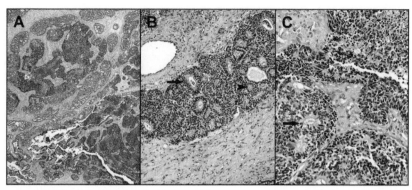

Fig. 2. Characteristic histologic features of higher grade ENB seen at (*A*) 2× magnification, (*B*) 10× magnification, and (*C*) 40× magnification with necrosis, increased mitotic activity and predominance of true-lumen, Flexner-Wintersteiner rosettes (*arrows*). Homer-Wright pseudorosettes (*arrowhead*) are more frequently seen in low-grade ENB. See Hyams' grading system (see **Table 2**).

Table 1
Immunohistochemical profile for ENB

Marker	Pattern	Diagnostic Significance
Neuron-Specific Enolase	Diffusely positive	Characteristic of ENB
Synaptophysin	Diffusely positive	Characteristic of ENB
Chromogranin	Often positive	Characteristic of ENB
Cytokeratin	Variable	Characteristically positive in SNUC, punctuate paranuclear positivity in SNNEC
Glial Fibrillary Acidic Protein	Variable	—
Neurofibrillary Protein	Variable	—
β-tubulin	Variable	—
Microtubule-Associated Protein	Variable	—
Epithelial Membrane Antigen	Variable	—
Leu-7 (CD57)	Variable	—
CD56	Variable	—
CD57	Variable	—
AE1/AE3	Variable	—
S-100	Variable, in peripheral Schwann-like cells	Sinonasal melanoma will be diffusely positive
HMB-45	Variable, and focal	Sinonasal melanoma will be diffusely positive
Common Leukocyte Antigen	Negative	Sinonasal lymphoma will be positive
Desmin	Negative	Rhabdomyosarcoma will be positive
Myogenin	Negative	Rhabdomyosarcoma will be positive
Vimentin	Negative	Rhabdomyosarcoma will be positive
Actin	Negative	Rhabdomyosarcoma will be positive
MIC2 (CD99)	Negative	PNET/EWS will be positive
FLI1	Negative	PNET/EWS will be positive
Pituitary Adenoma Hormones • GH, PRL, Corticotropin, TSH, FSH/LH • Glycoprotein hormone alpha subunit	Negative	Pituitary adenoma variably positive

Abbreviations: FSH/LH, follicle-stimulating hormone and luteinizing hormone; GH, growth hormone; PNET/EWS, peripheral neuroectodermal tumor and Ewing sarcoma; PRL, prolactin; SNNEC, sinonasal neuroendocrine carcinoma; SNUC, sinonasal undifferentiated carcinoma; TSH, thyroid stimulating hormone.

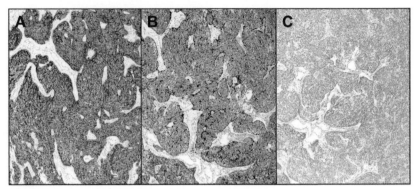

Fig. 3. Characteristic immunohistochemical staining of ENB. (*A*) Synaptophysin is diffusely positive. (*B*) S-100 highlights sustentacular cells. (*C*) Cytokeratin cocktail is negative.

a biopsy.[9] Additionally, poorly differentiated tumors can be difficult to distinguish from other, more aggressive, tumors that are associated with a worse outcome than ENB.[21]

DIFFERENTIAL DIAGNOSIS

The differential diagnosis for ENB is extremely broad. ENB must be considered whenever a sinonasal mass lesion is identified. In particular, ENB can be confused histologically with several other "round cell tumors" of the nasal cavity and paranasal sinuses.[18] **Box 1** presents several diagnoses that must be considered in the differential when an ENB is encountered. Tumors commonly confused with ENB include sinonasal undifferentiated carcinoma, sinonasal neuroendocrine carcinoma, small cell carcinoma, pituitary adenoma, melanoma, lymphoma, and rhabdomyosarcoma. Careful pathologic review and accurate immunohistochemical analysis are essential, and the typical differentiating characteristics are summarized above. The behavior of ENB compared with non-ENB neuroendocrine tumors differs greatly, with non-ENB tumors posing a greater risk of regional and distant

failure.[21] Thus, the approach to treatment of these two entities also differs greatly. Optimal outcomes are achieved when systemic therapy is used for non-ENB neuroendocrine tumors, whereas ENB is often controlled with local therapy alone (most often, surgery with postoperative irradiation).[21] Thus, differentiating ENB from these other entities is essential. Characteristic histologic findings and immunohistochemical staining patterns in ENB are summarized in **Table 1**. Differentiating ENB from other neuroendocrine entities can be difficult. Histologically, sinonasal undifferentiated carcinoma (SNUC) and neuroendocrine carcinoma (NEC) tend to have a higher mitotic rate and show areas of necrosis. Immunohistochemistry will be positive for cytokeratin, whereas ENB is characteristically negative. S-100 stains sustentacular cells in ENB, but is characteristically absent in SNUC and NEC.[18,22,23]

STAGING SYSTEMS

As with any malignancy, once the diagnosis of ENB is established and the proper diagnostic workup has been obtained, it is necessary to stage

Table 2				
Grading scale according to Hyams				
Grade	**1**	**2**	**3**	**4**
Architecture	Lobular	Lobular	Variable	Variable
Mitotic activity	Absent	Present	Prominent	Marked
Nuclear pleomorphism	Absent	Moderate	Prominent	Marked
Fibrillary matrix	Prominent	Present	Minimal	Absent
Rosettes	HW	HW	FW	FW
Necrosis	Absent	Absent	+/− Present	Common

Abbreviations: FW, Flexner-Wintersteiner; HW, Homer-Wright.

Data from Hyams VJ. Olfactory neuroblastoma. In: Hyams VJ, BJ, Michaels L, editors. Tumors of the upper respiratory tract and ear. Washington, DC: Armed Forces Institute of Pathology; 1988. p. 240–8.

Box 1
Differential diagnosis for ENB

Malignant neoplasms

Round cell tumors

ENB

Sinonasal undifferentiated carcinoma

Sinonasal neuroendocrine carcinoma

Sinonasal malignant melanoma

Small cell undifferentiated (neuroendo-crine) carcinoma

Undifferentiated (lymphoepithelioma-like) carcinoma

Extraosseous Ewing sarcoma/PNET

Rhabdomyosarcoma

Mesenchymal chondrosarcoma

Small cell osteosarcoma

Synovial sarcoma

Natural killer/T-cell lymphoma

Extramedullary plasmacytoma

Other histologies

Sinonasal squamous cell carcinoma

Adenocarcinoma

Adenoid cystic carcinoma

Nasopharyngeal carcinoma

Osteosarcoma

Chondrosarcoma

Benign neoplasms

Inverting papilloma

Pituitary adenoma

Congenital lesion

Dermoid

Encephalocele

Glioma

Infectious or inflammatory

Inflammatory polyps

Allergic fungal sinusitis

Sarcoidosis

divided into those that involve the nasal cavity alone (Kadish A), those extending to the paranasal sinuses (Kadish B), and those that extend outside of the paranasal sinuses (Kadish C)[24] (**Box 2**A). Noting that this system does not incorporate regional or distant metastasis, Morita and colleagues[25] modified the Kadish classification system in 1993, designating class D as those with metastases, which includes regional nodal disease and distant metastasis (see **Box 2**B). The classification system proposed by Dulguerov and colleagues[13] separates those patients with and without sphenoid sinus disease, as well as differentiates between those with intracranial and/or orbital extension from those with brain parenchymal invasion. This system also considers lymph node and distant metastasis separately (see **Box 2**C). A classification system proposed by Biller and colleagues[26] is perhaps the most detailed, differentiating between those tumors with extension to the brain that are amenable to surgery, and those that are not. It also segregates those with lymph node and distant metastases (see **Box 2**D). The TNM staging system for paranasal sinus tumors as described by the American Joint Committee on Cancer[27] can also be applied; however, the biologic behavior unique to ENB compared with other sinonasal tumors, makes the above-mentioned classification systems more applicable to this disease.

There remains debate as to which staging system is most appropriate and useful for the evaluation and treatment planning in ENB. Each of the factors emphasized by the different systems is important to consider when determining the surgical approach or options, the benefit of adjuvant treatments, and the overall prognosis of the patient. What seems clear is that there is a distinct difference in prognosis between those patients who present with metastatic disease and those who do not, and the authors recommend routine use of a system that considers nodal and distant metastasis. A review of the SEER database showed significant differences in outcome between the four groups when modified Kadish classification was applied. Also, there was a strong association between poor disease-specific survival and the presence of lymph node metastsis.[7] In their meta-analysis, Dulguerov and colleagues[3] also showed that lymph node metastasis was associated with a poor prognosis. The study by Zafereo and colleagues[14] found that the Dulguerov system or a TNM-based staging separated those patients with worse disease-free survival, whereas the Kadish system did not. Another large single-institution study noted that both the Kadish and Dulguerov system could

the cancer to make treatment decisions and provide prognostic information. There have been several staging systems proposed for this disease and no single system has become universally accepted. The first staging system created, and the most commonly applied, was proposed by Kadish and colleagues[24] in 1976. This staging system classifies local disease only, and is simply

---

Box 2
Staging systems proposed for ENB

Systems proposed by (A) Kadish (B) Morita (C) Dulguerov and (D) Biller

A. Kadish stages

   A. Tumor confined to the nasal cavity

   B. Tumor involvement of the nasal cavity and paranasal sinuses

   C. Tumor extends beyond the nasal cavity and paranasal sinuses

B. Morita modification

   A. Tumor confined to the nasal cavity

   B. Tumor involvement of the nasal cavity and paranasal sinuses

   C. Tumor extends beyond the nasal cavity and paranasal sinuses

   D. Presence of metastases (regional or distant)

C. Dulguerov staging system

   T1. Tumor involves the nasal cavity and/or paranasal sinuses, but spares the sphenoid sinus and superior ethmoid cells

   T2. Tumor involves the sphenoid sinus and/or the cribriform plate

   T3. Tumor extends into the orbit or into the anterior cranial fossa, without invasion of the dura

   T4. Tumor involves the brain

   N0. No regional lymph node metastases

   N1. Lymph node metastases present

   M0. No distant metastases

   M1. Lymph node metastases present

D. Biller staging system

   T1. Tumor involves the nasal cavity/paranasal sinuses (excludes the sphenoid)

   T2. Extension into the orbit and/or cranial cavity

   T3. Brain involvement but deemed resectable

   T4. Extensive brain involvement, unresectable tumor

   N0. No regional lymph node metastases

   N1. Lymph node metastases present

   M0. No distant metastases

   M1. Lymph node metastases present

---

identify those patients at highest risk of local-regional recurrence[8] and supported the use of the latter system because it considers the presence of metastasis and the extent of local invasion, making it more informative.

The following sections describe the treatment and outcomes for patients with ENB. Outcomes are generally favorable, although ENB will recur in a significant number of patients, often after several years without evidence of disease. Optimal treatment regimens are still under investigation and there have been several recent advances that have potentially improved treatment and decreased morbidity, namely the applications of endoscopic surgery and intensity-modulated radiation therapy (IMRT). That there is not yet a universally accepted staging system is largely due to the evolution of the standard of care for ENB and the long follow-up necessary to compare outcomes among patients with this rare disease, making it difficult to assess which staging system is most useful.

TREATMENT

There are three modalities used to treat ENB: surgery, external beam radiation, and chemotherapy. Often, a combination of these modalities is used, namely surgical resection with postoperative irradiation, for all but the smallest tumors. Chemotherapy has a role for more advanced cases, but the utility of chemotherapeutic agents is not well-defined. A detailed review of each modality follows.

Surgical Approaches

It has largely been established that the mainstay treatment of ENB is complete surgical resection. ENB arises in a region in close proximity to the structures of the orbit and anterior skull base. Preservation of these structures when they are not involved, and resection of these structures when there is clear invasion, adds to the complexity of the surgical approaches for these tumors. Also, the proximity of these structures makes it difficult to obtain wide resection with clear margins. Craniotomy can potentially be avoided if preoperative imaging clearly shows that the cribriform plate and superior ethmoid air cells are free of disease, but this is very rare. Otherwise, a craniofacial resection approach has been advocated as the standard of care.

The traditional and standard approach to resection of ENB is anterior craniofacial resection, involving a bifrontal craniotomy combined with a transfacial approach, through either a lateral rhinotomy incision or a Weber-Ferguson facial flap for increased exposure (**Fig. 4**). Craniotomy is usually performed via a bicoronal scalp incision with preservation of the pericranium pedicled anteriorly, which can be turned into the defect to eliminate the communication between the intracranial space and the nasal cavity after resection. Burr holes are created and the bifrontal craniotomy is performed with preservation of the underlying dura. The frontal lobes are allowed to relax back to expose the anterior skull base, olfactory region, and the ENB. The anterior craniofacial approach and resection are depicted in **Fig. 5**. All tumors which reach the skull base (Kadish B and C) require dural resection and resection of the olfactory tracts. It is typically not possible to successfully resect the tumor and preserve olfaction; even for unilateral disease. Intracerebral invasion is managed by focal cerebral resection. A margin of a millimeter or two is all that is necessary in the brain. Dural extension must be pursued to negative margins. Dural closure is performed under the operating microscope and should be watertight. Primary closure is usually not possible and dural grafting is typically required. Reconstruction of the floor of the anterior cranial fossa is achieved by rotating in a vascularized pericranial graft. The graft is sutured to the residual bone of the central skull base and/or the dura distal to the site of dural grafting.

With anterior craniofacial resection, the tumor is also inferiorly approached, and the traditional open techniques require a lateral rhinotomy or Weber-Ferguson incision. If the nasal component of the tumor is limited to the midline nasal cavity, a lateral rhinotomy incision with transnasal approach may be sufficient. A lip-split with a gingivobuccal incision can be added for increased exposure and access if necessary. As more lateral exposure is necessary, the Weber-Ferguson facial flap can be used. Another, less commonly used, approach is the facial degloving procedure, which avoids incisions on the face, but can distort the nasal anatomy because the lower lateral cartilages

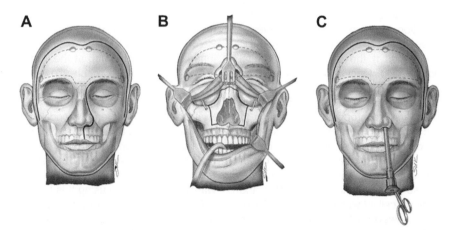

A   **B**   **C**

Fig. 4. Transfacial approaches for anterior craniofacial resection. (*A*) Lateral rhinotomy incision combined with lip-splitting incision to create the Weber-Ferguson flap. (*B*) Facial degloving approach. (*C*) Endoscopic approach can circumvent facial incisions in selected cases. (*From* Department of Head and Neck Surgery and Department of Neurosurgery, The University of Texas M.D. Anderson Cancer Center; with permission.)

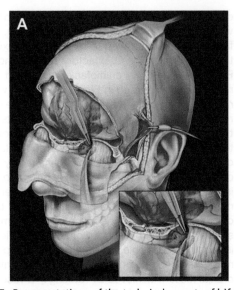
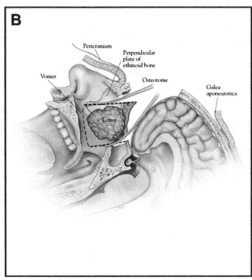

Fig. 5. Representations of the technical aspects of bifrontal craniotomy during anterior craniofacial resection. (*A*) A bicoronal incision is made, the pericranium is preserved and reflected anteriorly. Bifrontal craniotomy is performed and care is taken to preserve the dura. Inset shows reflection of the periorbita if necessary with control of the ethmoidal arterial system. (*B*) The frontal lobes are allowed to relax to expose the anterior skull base, and resection is performed with inferior exposure and tumor clearance via a transfacial or endoscopic approach. (*From* Department of Head and Neck Surgery and Department of Neurosurgery, The University of Texas M.D. Anderson Cancer Center; with permission.)

are disarticulated from the upper lateral cartilages and the nasal soft tissues are reflected superiorly. The exposure with this approach is also arguably more limited (see **Fig. 4**).

The lateral resection can range from medial maxillectomy, to subtotal, or even total, maxillectomy with or without orbital exenteration. The extent of resection necessary depends on the involvement of the tumor. Removal of portions of the bony maxilla, particularly the medial wall (eg, the lateral nasal wall, middle turbinate, and inferior turbinate), is often necessary to gain adequate exposure for complete resection of the midline tumor, even if these structures are not directly involved. The orbit can often be spared if the periorbita or orbital septum is not invaded. Once tumor has involved the orbital fat, extraocular muscles, or other intraorbital contents, the eye cannot be saved. Even if the globe can be spared, postoperative irradiation to the orbit often renders the eye nonfunctional with significant xerophthalmia after irradiation of the lacrimal system. Thus, exenteration provides better tumor control with a more satisfactory functional outcome in these cases. Tumor control rates and survival are often excellent with the anterior craniofacial approach; however, other approaches have been sought to limit both frontal lobe retraction and to eliminate facial scars.

The transglabellar-subcranial resection was first described by Raveh and colleagues[28] in 1988. This approach is executed via the bicoronal incision alone. The pericranial flap is preserved and the frontal craniotomy is performed. The transglabellar-subcranial modification places the inferior cuts of the craniotomy lower across the nasal bridge and superior orbital rims. The extent of superior orbital rim, frontal bone, and nasal bridge that is resected depends on tumor size, location, and exposure necessary for complete removal with negative margins. The distal 3 to 5 mm of nasal bone is preserved to maintain the internal nasal valve. To remove the bone flap, it must be fractured from the crista galli and nasal septum. Before removal of the flap, fixation plates are fashioned to replace the flap at the end of the procedure. This direct approach allows exposure and resection of the anterior skull base, with less retraction of the frontal lobes, but somewhat limited exposure inferiorly and posteriorly. The pericranial flap is turned inward to close the superior nasal cavity at the end of the procedure and the bony flap is replaced. Ward and colleagues[15] have recently reported a series of 15 patients with good outcomes using this technique.

Endoscopic surgery in the nasal cavity and paranasal sinuses has advanced significantly in the last two decades. Endoscopic-assisted craniofacial resection, as well as a purely transnasal endoscopic approach, has been advocated for carefully selected cases of ENB.[29–32] The endoscopic approaches completely avoid facial incisions and alteration of the bony facial anatomy. Endoscopic resection can be performed via a purely transnasal approach or with the addition of a gingival-buccal, transmaxillary (Caldwell-Luc) approach for added exposure. To accomplish the endoscopic approach, the tumor is typically debulked in a systematic fashion to identify and preserve the root of the tumor (often the skull base at the superior nasal cavity for ENB). Then, uninvolved structures surrounding the tumor are resected or widely opened to provide exposure (eg, medial maxillectomy, sphenoid sinus, frontal sinuses). Vascular control of the feeding vessels to the tumor, for example from the anterior ethmoidal or sphenopalatine arteries, is obtained. The bony skull base surrounding the lesion is then exposed and, subsequently, opened. Tumor with surrounding bone, dura, or brain parenchyma can then be removed, either via the craniotomy approach or endoscopically. Steps from the purely endoscopic technique are shown in **Fig. 6**. Pinheiro-Neto and colleagues[12] provide an excellent detailed review of the technical aspects involved with the endoscopic approach to tumors of the anterior skull base. The authors have more often used endoscopic-assisted craniofacial resection for ENB, but have recently used the purely endoscopic approach for small tumors without extensive dural invasion. Early reports describing results of endoscopic resection have been favorable,[29,32] but large series with adequate long-term follow-up will be necessary to prove that these techniques are truly comparable to traditional resection for patients with ENB.

There is debate about appropriate management of the cervical lymph nodes for patients with ENB. Reports have varied greatly in the incidence of cervical lymph node metastases at the time of presentation to, as well as after, initial treatment. The incidence of cervical lymph node involvement at the time of presentation is likely 5% to 8%, but the incidence of the eventual development of neck disease is likely 20% to 25% (it should be noted that the cervical lymph nodes are often untreated previous to metastasis, in these cases).[17] Despite this relatively high rate, surgical management of the neck is generally reserved for patients who present with clinical or radiographic evidence of disease, or for those who develop lymph node metastases after treatment at the primary site. There are no reports indicating that elective or prophylactic neck dissection is beneficial, and an elective surgical approach has not generally been advocated. However, in current practice, the neck is often irradiated electively as part of the postoperative radiation plan. The extent of neck dissection when lymph node disease is present is tailored to the neck levels involved with disease, and a selective or functional approach is generally favored if this technique allows complete resection of known disease. Postoperative irradiation is advocated[33] and the role of concurrent chemotherapy is unclear.

Radiation Therapy

Radiation is an important treatment modality in the management of ENB, but the optimal use of this modality is not entirely clear. Radiation can be

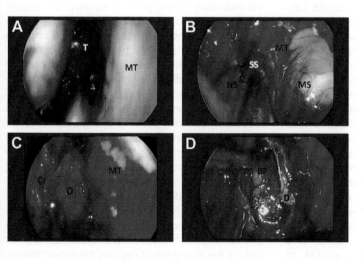

Fig. 6. Technical approach to endoscopic or endoscopic-assisted resection. (A) Tumor is debulked and origin identified (MT, middle turbinate; T, tumor). (B) Surrounding normal structures are resected or opened to provide exposure—the sphenoid and posterior ethmoid sinuses are opened to establish the level of the skull base and safely dissect from posterior to anterior (MS, opened maxillary sinus; SS, opened sphenoid sinus; MT, root of resected middle turbinate; NS, nasal septum). (C) The involved bony skull base is resected and the underlying dura is exposed (Cr, cribriform plate, containing olfactory rootlets near the superior attachment of the nasal septum; D, dura; MT, root of resected middle turbinate). (D) The underlying dura is resected with clear margins (BP, brain parenchyma; D, dura). (From Department of Head and Neck Surgery, The University of Texas M.D. Anderson Cancer Center; with permission.)

delivered as the primary modality of treatment, or in the preoperative or postoperative setting. The most common and most widely accepted method is postoperative radiotherapy delivered after definitive resection.

Irradiation as a primary mode of treatment has been used in the past, but several studies have demonstrated that surgery combined with irradiation is superior to irradiation used as definitive therapy.[3,7,32,34] Irradiation may be used alone or in combination with concurrent chemotherapy when surgical resection is not an option. This may be due to local or metastatic tumor involvement rendering complete resection impossible or if surgery is not an option due to medical contraindications. Radiation treatment at this time is typically delivered using IMRT, which provides optimal sparing of radiation dose to sensitive normal structures, such as the optic nerve or brain. Gross tumor is typically treated with 1.8 to 2 Gy fractions up to a total dose of 65 to 70 Gy.

The widely accepted role for radiation treatment is in the postoperative setting. Postoperative radiation therapy (PORT) is typically delivered in 2 Gy fractions up to a total dose of approximately 60 Gy, with the goal of treating microscopic residual disease and reduction of the rate of local-regional recurrence. The authors again advocate the use of IMRT to optimize off-target dosing. Reports limited to relatively small series and the lack of controlled, prospective analysis has made it difficult to demonstrate a clear advantage of surgery and irradiation over complete surgical resection alone. However, several large reviews show a trend toward improved survival with PORT[3,7] and several published series support this approach[15,35] (Ow TJ, Hanna EY, Roberts DB, et al. Multimodality therapy optimizes long-term outcome in patients with esthesioneuroblastoma. Unpublished data, manuscript under review, 2012).

Another potential strategy is to give radiation therapy in the preoperative setting. The theoretical advantages of this method are improved accuracy in delineating the target volume with improved sparing of adjacent critical structures, and less anticipated local hypoxia secondary to postsurgical changes. Preoperative radiation may potentially reduce tumor volume improving the respectability of large tumors.[36] However, the target lesion may also become less defined at the time of resection. A well-described protocol using preoperative irradiation or chemoradiation has been reported by the group at University of Virginia.[36,37] Bachar and colleagues[8] recently reported on a subset of patients treated with a preoperative irradiation approach and there were no clear differences in survival or recurrence identified when these

patients were compared with those that received PORT in their series; however, these subgroups were small.

The data regarding elective irradiation of the neck parallel the paucity of data examining prophylactic neck dissection. Ozashin and colleagues[34] reported only a 7% rate of regional relapse when the neck was not irradiated, and Noh and colleagues[17] did not find that elective irradiation prevented regional failure. Other studies suggest that the development of regional disease is much higher over time, and there is some limited data providing support for elective irradiation of the cervical lymph nodes.[38] Currently, it remains unresolved if there is an advantage to elective irradiation of the neck, though this is commonly employed.

The recent utility of proton beam irradiation, particularly intensity-modulated proton beam radiation therapy (IMPBRT) deserves mention. This technique allows delivery of therapeutic-dose radiation to a target while minimizing the dose to the surrounding, uninvolved structures. There has been preliminary data using this technique in ENB,[39] and this modality may prove to be ideally suited for skull base malignancies.[40] Future studies are necessary to establish the role of IMPBRT in ENB, but this technique offers a promising option in the management of tumors of the skull base.

Chemotherapy

The data supporting chemotherapy for the treatment of ENB is limited. Chemotherapy as a single modality is reserved for palliation. Chemotherapeutic regimens are otherwise generally used in the induction setting prior to surgery, or concurrently with postoperative radiation. At our institution, neoadjuvant regimens often include cisplatin and etoposide, and are typically advocated for those patients with advanced disease, particularly those with significant intracranial or orbital invasion. We also advocate concurrent chemoradiation with platinum-based treatment after surgical resection for those patients at high risk of local-regional recurrence. This decision is not based on strong data in treating ENB, and is empirically extrapolated from the current practices in treating other head and neck malignancies.[41]

Data specifically examining the utility of chemotherapy for ENB is limited to case reports and small series. Interestingly, in a series published by Noh and colleagues,[42] elective neck irradiation did not reduce the incidence of regional treatment failure, whereas none of the patients who received systemic chemotherapy recurred in the cervical lymph nodes. Chao and colleagues[43] reported on

8 patients who received neoadjuvant chemo-therapy (four received a cyclophosphamide/vincristine-based regimen, and 4 received cisplatin and etoposide), 6 of whom were NED at the time the study was completed. Two cases of preopera-tive chemoradiation with cisplatin and etoposide were detailed by Sohrabi and colleagues,[44] offering another potential treatment strategy em-ploying chemotherapy for patients with advanced ENB. Neoadjuvant chemotherapy was also sup-ported in a study of ifosfamide, cisplatin, and eto-poside, in which nine of eleven patients achieved an objective response with this regimen.[45] Perhaps the most well-studied chemotherapy protocol has been the regimen developed at the University of Virginia, which advocates concurrent administra-tion of cyclophosphamide and vincristine during preoperative irradiation.[37] A case of a durable response to sunitinib (a multi-kinase inhibitor that targets PDGFR, VEGFR, and KIT) in the palliative setting has also been published, offering another intriguing option for study in the era of targeted therapy.[46]

Summary of Treatment Strategies for ENB

Single-modality treatment of ENB is generally reserved for small tumors with no sign of regional or distant metastasis, and surgical resection is advocated. As disease becomes more locally advanced, more extensive surgery–typically an open or endoscopic-assisted craniofacial resec-tion is advocated, along with post-operative radia-tion therapy. Preoperative radiation is an alternative strategy which may yield equivalent results, and induction chemotherapy, as well as concurrent post-operative chemoradiation may improve local, regional, and distant control. Treat-ment of the neck is reserved for those who present with or develop regional disease, and neck dissec-tion with postoperative radiation or chemoradiation is advocated. Patients with distant disease can be treated palliatively. Systemic treatment is war-ranted, and surgery or irradiation for the primary site of disease may be considered. Chemoradia-tion is an approach for patients with unresectable local disease, which could subsequently improve the resectability for locally-advanced ENB.

PROGNOSIS AND FOLLOW-UP

Patients with ENB, even those with advanced local disease, often have an extended disease-free period, with a substantial number of patients demonstrating no evidence of disease after 10 to 15 years of follow-up. Recurrence can manifest late, often between 5–10 years after initial treat-ment[8,32,34,47,48] (Ow TJ, Hanna EY, Roberts DB,

et al. Multimodality therapy optimizes long-term outcome in patients with esthesioneuroblastoma. Unpublished data, manuscript under review, 2012). Close, long-term follow-up is mandatory for patients with ENB, typically with clinical exam, nasal endoscopy, and anatomic imaging. The authors advocate examination every 3–6 months with CT scan and/or MRI for surveillance for a period of 2 years, which can be extended to 6–12 months afterward for a period of 10 years, or indefinitely. Surveillance for distant metastatic disease is warranted for those patients with advanced local disease, and certainly for those who present with or develop regional disease. We advocate yearly chest radiographs and liver func-tion tests, and/or fluorodeoxyglucose-positron emission tomography (FDG-PET) imaging for distant surveillance.

Several large series with long follow-up have re-ported a median time to recurrence or progression between 57–110 months,[8,34,47] and 10-year disease/recurrence-free survival rates in the range of roughly 50%–70%.[8,47] The meta-analysis by Dulguerov and colleagues[3] reviewed five studies that reported an average 10-year disease-free survival rate of 52%. It seems that, despite good long-term overall survival, recurrences are rela-tively high (approximately 50%) and can be most often expected to occur between 5 to 10 years after treatment. In a review of patients at the authors' institution, despite excellent survival outcomes (disease-specific survival of 11.6 years), 46% of patients eventually developed recurrent disease, with a median time to recurrence of 6.9 years (Ow TJ, Hanna EY, Roberts DB, et al. Multimodality therapy optimizes long-term outcome in patients with esthesioneuroblastoma. Unpublished data, manuscript under review, 2012).

From the existing literature, it seems that patients with ENB are at risk of local, regional, and distant recurrence during follow-up. In the large series by Bachar and colleagues,[8] local, regional, and distant failure rates were observed at 15%, 18%, and 8%, respectively. Ozsahin and colleagues[34] reported higher overall local, regional, and distant failure rates, reporting 31%, 26%, and 19%, respectively. In their meta-analysis, Dulguerov and colleagues[3] reported that local, regional, and distant failure was 29%, 16%, and 17%, respectively. Review of the authors' experience showed that the site of first recurrence was local in 18% patients, regional in 18% of patients, and at distant sites in 10%. Distant failure was intracranial, pericranial, or spinal in 10 of 12 sites recorded (Ow TJ, Hanna EY, Roberts DB, et al. Multimodality therapy optimizes long-term outcome in patients with esthesioneuroblastoma. Unpublished data, manuscript under review,

2012). It seems that patients are at relatively high risk for local-regional failure (perhaps 30%–40%) when followed for an extended period. However, distant failure also remains a concern, with an approximate long-term risk of 10%–20%.

There are no data to advocate an optimal approach to treat recurrent disease, but aggressive salvage treatment seems warranted when feasible. Local or regional recurrence should be treated with surgical salvage when disease is resectable. If local or regional sites have not been previously irradiated, radiation or chemoradiation can be used either postoperatively or as a primary salvage modality in unresectable patients. Due to the long disease-free intervals seen among patients with ENB, re-irradiation may be an option in the salvage setting, but this has not been studied.

CURRENT CONTROVERSIES AND FUTURE DIRECTIONS

The diagnosis and management of ENB has improved significantly in the last three decades, yet several important questions remain unanswered. Because the recurrence patterns of this disease are better described with long-term studies of large patient sets, it will become more clear which staging system is most accurate and useful for guiding treatment and for prognostication. Perhaps further molecular and genetic evaluation will be added to the diagnostic work-up to improve our ability to accurately discriminate ENBs that are poorly differentiated from other entities. IMRT and endoscopic surgery have decreased morbidity with treatment, but well-planned, multi-institutional prospective studies will be necessary to determine if new therapies are equivalent or better than current standards. Also, given the fairly high rate of early and late regional metastases that have been recently reported and the prognostic implications of regional disease, it seems that proper management of the neck during treatment and follow-up should be scrutinized. These studies will be crucial to the refinement of the multimodality approach to treating this rare disease. As the array of chemotherapeutics exponentially increases, molecular targets must be sought to further tailor strategies to treat ENB, especially in the cases of locoregionally advanced, recurrent, and distantly metastatic disease.

REFERENCES

1. Berger L, LG, Richard D. L'esthesioneuroepitheliome olfactif. Bull Assoc Franc Etude Cancer 1924;13:410–2.
2. Broich G, Pagliari A, Ottaviani F. Esthesioneuroblastoma: a general review of the cases published since the discovery of the tumour in 1924. Anticancer Res 1997;17(4A):2683–706.
3. Dulguerov P, Allal AS, Calcaterra TC. Esthesioneuroblastoma: a meta-analysis and review. Lancet Oncol 2001;2(11):683–90.
4. Carney ME, O'Reilly RC, Sholevar B, et al. Expression of the human Achaete-scute 1 gene in olfactory neuroblastoma (esthesioneuroblastoma). J Neurooncol 1995;26(1):35–43.
5. Franssen EH, de Bree FM, Verhaagen J. Olfactory ensheathing glia: their contribution to primary olfactory nervous system regeneration and their regenerative potential following transplantation into the injured spinal cord. Brain Res Rev 2007;56(1):236–58.
6. Trojanowski JQ, Lee V, Pillsbury N, et al. Neuronal origin of human esthesioneuroblastoma demonstrated with anti-neurofilament monoclonal antibodies. N Engl J Med 1982;307(3):159–61.
7. Jethanamest D, Morris LG, Sikora AG, et al. Esthesioneuroblastoma: a population-based analysis of survival and prognostic factors. Arch Otolaryngol Head Neck Surg 2007;133(3):276–80.
8. Bachar G, Goldstein DP, Shah M, et al. Esthesioneuroblastoma: The Princess Margaret Hospital experience. Head Neck 2008;30(12):1607–14.
9. Platek ME, Merzianu M, Mashtare TL, et al. Improved survival following surgery and radiation therapy for olfactory neuroblastoma: analysis of the SEER database. Radiat Oncol 2011;6:41.
10. Klepin HD, McMullen KP, Lesser GJ. Esthesioneuroblastoma. Curr Treat Options Oncol 2005;6(6):509–18.
11. Rhoton AL Jr. The anterior and middle cranial base. Neurosurgery 2002;51(Suppl 4):S273–302.
12. Pinheiro-Neto CD, Fernandez-Miranda JC, Wang EW, et al. Anatomical correlates of endonasal surgery for sinonasal malignancies. Clin Anat 2012;25(1):129–34.
13. Dulguerov P, Calcaterra T. Esthesioneuroblastoma: the UCLA experience 1970–1990. Laryngoscope 1992;102(8):843–9.
14. Zafereo ME, Fakhri S, Prayson R, et al. Esthesioneuroblastoma: 25-year experience at a single institution. Otolaryngol Head Neck Surg 2008;138(4):452–8.
15. Ward PD, Heth JA, Thompson BG, et al. Esthesioneuroblastoma: results and outcomes of a single Institution's experience. Skull Base 2009;19(2):133–40.
16. Yaman H, Alkan N, Yilmaz S, et al. Is routine histopathological analysis of nasal polyposis specimens necessary? Eur Arch Otorhinolaryngol 2011;268(7):1013–5.
17. Zanation AM, Ferlito A, Rinaldo A, et al. When, how and why to treat the neck in patients with esthesioneuroblastoma: a review. Eur Arch Otorhinolaryngol 2010;267(11):1667–71.
18. Iezzoni JC, Mills SE. "Undifferentiated" small round cell tumors of the sinonasal tract: differential

diagnosis update. Am J Clin Pathol 2005; 124(Suppl):S110–21.

19. Faragalla H, Weinreb I. Olfactory neuroblastoma: a review and update. Adv Anat Pathol 2009;16(5): 322–31.

20. Hyams VJ. Olfactory neuroblastoma. In: Hyams VJ, BJ, Michaels L, editors. Tumors of the upper respiratory tract and ear. Washington, DC: Armed Forces Institute of Pathology; 1988. p. 240–8.

21. Rosenthal DI, Barker JL Jr, El-Naggar AK, et al. Sinonasal malignancies with neuroendocrine differentiation: patterns of failure according to histologic phenotype. Cancer 2004;101(11):2567–73.

22. Cordes B, Williams MD, Tirado Y, et al. Molecular and phenotypic analysis of poorly differentiated sinonasal neoplasms: an integrated approach for early diagnosis and classification. Hum Pathol 2009;40(3):283–92.

23. Mitchell EH, Diaz A, Yilmaz T, et al. Multimodality treatment for sinonasal neuroendocrine carcinoma. Head Neck 2011.

24. Kadish S, Goodman M, Wang CC. Olfactory neuroblastoma. A clinical analysis of 17 cases. Cancer 1976;37(3):1571–6.

25. Morita A, Ebersold MJ, Olsen KD, et al. Esthesioneuroblastoma: prognosis and management. Neurosurgery 1993;32(5):706–14 [discussion: 14–5].

26. Biller HF, Lawson W, Sachdev VP, et al. Esthesioneuroblastoma: surgical treatment without radiation. Laryngoscope 1990;100(11):1199–201.

27. Edge SB, Byrd DR, Compton CC. AJCC cancer staging manual. New York, NY: Springer; 2010.

28. Raveh J, Vuillemin T, Sutter F. Subcranial management of 395 combined frontobasal-midface fractures. Arch Otolaryngol Head Neck Surg 1988;114(10):1114–22.

29. Hanna E, DeMonte F, Ibrahim S, et al. Endoscopic resection of sinonasal cancers with and without craniotomy: oncologic results. Arch Otolaryngol Head Neck Surg 2009;135(12):1219–24.

30. Gallia GL, Reh DD, Salmasi V, et al. Endonasal endoscopic resection of esthesioneuroblastoma: the Johns Hopkins Hospital experience and review of the literature. Neurosurg Rev 2011;34(4):465–75.

31. Castelnuovo PG, Delu G, Sberze F, et al. Esthesioneuroblastoma: endonasal endoscopic treatment. Skull Base 2006;16(1):25–30.

32. Devaiah AK, Andreoli MT. Treatment of esthesioneuroblastoma: a 16-year meta-analysis of 361 patients. Laryngoscope 2009;119(7):1412–6.

33. Gore MR, Zanation AM. Salvage treatment of late neck metastasis in esthesioneuroblastoma: a meta-analysis. Arch Otolaryngol Head Neck Surg 2009; 135(10):1030–4.

34. Ozsahin M, Gruber G, Olszyk O, et al. Outcome and prognostic factors in olfactory neuroblastoma: a rare cancer network study. Int J Radiat Oncol Biol Phys 2010;78(4):992–7.

35. Foote RL, Morita A, Ebersold MJ, et al. Esthesioneuroblastoma: the role of adjuvant radiation therapy. Int J Radiat Oncol Biol Phys 1993;27(4):835–42.

36. Eden BV, Debo RF, Larner JM, et al. Esthesioneuroblastoma. Long-term outcome and patterns of failure—the University of Virginia experience. Cancer 1994;73(10):2556–62.

37. Sheehan JM, Sheehan JP, Jane JA Sr, et al. Chemotherapy for esthesioneuroblastomas. Neurosurg Clin N Am 2000;11(4):693–701.

38. Monroe AT, Hinerman RW, Amdur RJ, et al. Radiation therapy for esthesioneuroblastoma: rationale for elective neck irradiation. Head Neck 2003;25(7):529–34.

39. Nishimura H, Ogino T, Kawashima M, et al. Proton-beam therapy for olfactory neuroblastoma. Int J Radiat Oncol Biol Phys 2007;68(3):758–62.

40. Frank SJ, Selek U. Proton beam radiation therapy for head and neck malignancies. Curr Oncol Rep 2010; 12(3):202–7.

41. Bernier J, Cooper JS, Pajak TF, et al. Defining risk levels in locally advanced head and neck cancers: a comparative analysis of concurrent postoperative radiation plus chemotherapy trials of the EORTC (#22931) and RTOG (# 9501). Head Neck 2005; 27(10):843–50.

42. Noh OK, Lee SW, Yoon SM, et al. Radiotherapy for esthesioneuroblastoma: is elective nodal irradiation warranted in the multimodality treatment approach? Int J Radiat Oncol Biol Phys 2011;79(2):443–9.

43. Chao KS, Kaplan C, Simpson JR, et al. Esthesioneuroblastoma: the impact of treatment modality. Head Neck 2001;23(9):749–57.

44. Sohrabi S, Drabick JJ, Crist H, et al. Neoadjuvant concurrent chemoradiation for advanced esthesioneuroblastoma: a case series and review of the literature. J Clin Oncol 2011;29(13):e358–61.

45. Kim DW, Jo YH, Kim JH, et al. Neoadjuvant etoposide, ifosfamide, and cisplatin for the treatment of olfactory neuroblastoma. Cancer 2004;101(10): 2257–60.

46. Preusser M, Hutterer M, Sohm M, et al. Disease stabilization of progressive olfactory neuroblastoma (esthesioneuroblastoma) under treatment with sunitinib mesylate. J Neurooncol 2010;97(2):305–8.

47. de Gabory L, Abdulkhaleq HM, Darrouzet V, et al. Long-term results of 28 esthesioneuroblastomas managed over 35 years. Head Neck 2011;33(1): 82–6.

48. Diaz EM Jr, Johnigan RH 3rd, Pero C, et al. Olfactory neuroblastoma: the 22-year experience at one comprehensive cancer center. Head Neck 2005; 27(2):138–49.

Head and Neck Sarcomas
Epidemiology, Pathology, and Management

James Paul O'Neill, MB, MRCSI, MBA, MD, MMSc, ORL-HNS[a],*,
Mark H. Bilsky, MD[b], Dennis Kraus, MD[c]

KEYWORDS

- Sarcoma • Surgery • Radiation • Chemotherapy • Grade • Margins • Size

KEY POINTS

- Malignant fibrous histiocytoma, osteosarcoma, fibrosarcoma, angiosarcoma, rhabdomyosarcoma, and liposarcoma are the most frequently reported sarcomas in the head and neck.
- Sarcomas that metastasize to lymph nodes are clear cell, rhabdomyosarcomas, epithelioid, angiosarcoma, and synovial sarcomas.
- Sarcoma surgery demands a significant respect for tumor and pseudocapsule margins in an effort to succeed in gross disease removal with free microscopic margins. This removal can be challenging in an anatomically confined region such as the head and neck.
- Distant metastases occur in approximately 25% to 30% at diagnosis or during follow-up. The common sites of metastases are lung, bone, central nervous system, and liver. Patients require yearly chest imaging for life.

INTRODUCTION

Head and neck sarcomas are a diverse group of cancers. According to the American Cancer Society, in 2010 10,520 new sarcomas were predicted to occur, with 3920 deaths. Head and neck sarcomas account for approximately 2% to 15% of all sarcomas, representing approximately 1% of head and neck malignancies.[1] Sarcomas are classified according to their tissue of origin, which can be bone or soft tissue, whether the tumor is high or low grade, and the anatomic subsite of presentation within the head and neck. There lies an 80:20 distribution between these mesenchymal sarcomas of soft-tissue origin and those of bone and cartilage lineage. The increased use of the immunohistochemistry and molecular oncology markers has furthered our ability to definitively subclassify sarcomas; however, 20% will still remain unclassified, highlighting the challenges that remain.

Malignant fibrous histiocytomas (MFH), osteosarcomas, rhabdomyosarcomas, angiosarcomas, synovial sarcomas, and Ewing sarcomas are all considered high-grade tumors. Conversely, dermatofibrosarcoma protuberans, atypical lipomatous tumor, and desmoid tumor are predominately low grade. Chondrosarcoma, fibrosarcoma, liposarcoma, leiomyosarcoma, neurogenic sarcoma, and hemangiopericytoma require individualized grade characterization.[2] Grade is a key prognostic indicator according to the American Joint Committee on Cancer Staging (AJCC). Five-year survival rates for patients with grade 1 sarcomas was 100% in

No financial disclosures.

[a] Department of Head and Neck Surgery, Memorial Sloan-Kettering Cancer Center, 1275 York Avenue, New York, NY 10065, USA; [b] Department of Neurosurgery, Memorial Sloan-Kettering Cancer Center, 1275 York Avenue, New York, NY 10065, USA; [c] New York Head and Neck Institute, North Shore-Long Island Jewish Health System, New York, NY, USA
* Corresponding author.
E-mail address: joneill@rcsi.ie

neurosurgery.theclinics.com

one series, compared with 64% for those with tumors of grades 2 and 3.[3]

Computed tomography (CT) and magnetic resonance imaging (MRI) offer 3-dimensional information for tumor locoregional extension, provide assessment of tissue composition (vascular vs avascular, solid vs liquid, fat vs cellular), and assist in successful biopsy and pathologic confirmation, surgical extirpation, and adjuvant radiotherapy planning. Superior soft-tissue resolution on MRI with multiplanar advances provides intimate anatomic information relevant in areas of complex anatomy such as the skull base. ^{18}F-labeled fluorodeoxyglucose (FDG) positron emission tomography (PET) scanning has been used clinically for tumor staging and restaging, monitoring treatment, and predicting prognosis. FDG PET has been found to be superior to conventional imaging in evaluating patients with the more common head and neck malignancies such as squamous cell carcinomas, lymphomas, and salivary gland cancers. PET scanning may also be superior to conventional imaging in staging of miscellaneous cancers of the head and neck, including melanomas, basal cell carcinomas, olfactory neuroblastomas, and sarcomas.[4–6]

Surgery is the primary mode of treatment. Adjuvant radiation therapy (RT) should be considered for patients with locally recurrent lesions and intermediate to high-grade tumors, and for those with close or positive margins. Patients with advanced, marginally resectable tumors should be considered for preoperative RT. Although the role of chemotherapy for head and neck soft-tissue sarcomas remains to be fully defined, adjuvant chemotherapy as a means to decrease the risk for disease recurrence in patients with localized soft-tissue sarcoma at diagnosis has been investigated. The majority of trials reported on have been hampered by patient heterogeneity, short follow-up, and low patient accrual.[7] Neoadjuvant chemotherapy is, however, a strategy used for high-grade sarcomas in many tertiary referral cancer centers.

Patients with unresectable disease have the worst prognosis, and are treated with RT alone or in combination with chemotherapy. It has been difficult to assess the efficacy of RT alone because of selection bias, but it is not considered as effective as surgery alone or combined with RT if used for tumors of similar stage.[8]

MALIGNANT FIBROUS HISTIOCYTOMA

In 1964 O'Brien and Stout[9] published the first article to describe MFH, which is now the most commonly diagnosed soft-tissue sarcoma in the head and neck. Most often MFH occurs in the extremities and the retroperitoneum, and is described as an undifferentiated high-grade pleomorphic sarcoma. This tumor largely presents in the fifth and sixth decades, contributes up to 40% of all sarcomas in the head and neck, and has a male to female predominance of 2:1. Women tend to present nearly a decade earlier. Three percent to 10% of all MFHs occur within the head and neck, with the majority of these occurring in the sinonasal tract. These tumors have a strong association with ionizing radiation exposure, most commonly used for a prior diagnosis of squamous cell carcinoma and lymphoma pathology.[2,10–13]

An MFH tumor is composed of an admixture of spindle-shaped fibroblastic tumor cells and bizarre mononuclear histiocytic tumor cells arranged in a storiform pattern with some multinucleated giant cells. Histopathologic differential of MFH includes anaplastic lymphoma, pleomorphic leiomyosarcoma, pleomorphic liposarcoma, malignant melanoma, malignant peripheral nerve sheath tumor, anaplastic carcinoma, malignant gliomas, or gliosarcoma.[14] There are 5 different histologic patterns of MFH: inflammatory, giant cell, myxoid, storiform-pleomorphic, and angiomatous. Immunopositivity for vimentin, α1-antichymotrypsin, and Ki-67 have been demonstrated in MFH and are of diagnostic importance. The tumor tissue should be immunonegative for S-100 protein and cytokeratins. Histiocytic markers CD68, α1-antichymotrypsin, and factor XIII are no longer used in the diagnosis of MFH, as immunoreactivity to these markers is nonspecific.[15]

Radiation-induced sarcoma tends to occur at the periphery of the radiation field, where the dose of radiation can permanently alter the cell's ability to perform routine repair tasks. To link past radiation exposure and sarcoma, the following criteria must apply. There must be a documented history of irradiation to the head and neck and the new malignancy arising within the irradiated field. The tumor must be histologically distinct from the original primary lesion, and the latency period between the radiation exposure and the development of the new malignancy must be 5 years or more. It is estimated that after head and neck radiotherapy, the incidence of radiation-induced sarcoma ranges from 0.03% to 2.2% in those surviving more than 5 years.[16] The threshold dose for radiation-induced sarcoma is unknown, but the increased risk seemingly correlates with increasing radiation dose.[17] Radiation-induced MFH carries a poor prognosis and accounts for almost 50% of radiation-associated soft-tissue sarcomas.[18] Overall survival from radiation-induced sarcoma ranges from 10% to 30% at 5 years.[19]

Surgery is the main treatment modality for MFH, with chemotherapy and radiation used in the adjuvant setting. The classic behavior of MFH is to recur locally, although rarely it metastasizes to regional lymphatics. Surgical resection for MFH requires wide field dissection with generous margins, and when possible the tumor is never grossly visualized at the resection margin. Of course this is sometimes not feasible, especially within anatomic constraints of the head and neck, but dedicated preoperative planning is essential for successful tumor extirpation and reconstruction of the operative deficit. Despite aggressive surgical management, positive margins are associated with an increase in local recurrence and distant disease. The role of chemotherapy as neoadjuvant or adjuvant therapy remains unproven, and our ability to perform a randomized trial is remote. Distant metastasis appears in one-third of all cases, and those cases mainly involve the lung, regional lymph nodes, liver, and bone.

Five-year overall, disease-free, and disease-specific survival rates are 55%, 44%, and 69%, respectively. The main negative prognostic variables for MFH include positive margins, tumors of the head and neck anatomic region, tumor size greater than 5 cm, and high stage.[20,21]

OSTEOSARCOMA

Osteosarcomas (OS) represent approximately 1% of head and neck cancers and fewer than 10% of all osteosarcomas (**Figs. 1–4**).[22,23] Male to female distributions are similar. Patients present with OS of the head and neck in the third and fourth decades, in contrast to OS of the extremities, which generally afflicts teenagers. There are 3 subdivisions of conventional OS: osteoblastic, chondroblastic, and fibroblastic. Most OS will demonstrate components of all 3 subdivisions. There are also many other OS variants including multifocal, telangiectatic, small cell, intraosseous well-differentiated, intracortical, periosteal, parosteal, high-grade surface, and extraosseous OS.

Predisposition to this tumor is related to deletion of chromosome 13q14, which inactivates the retinoblastoma gene, bone dysplasias such as Paget disease, fibrous dysplasia, and enchondromatosis. Li Fraumeni syndrome due to germline TP53 mutations predisposes to osteosarcoma and Rothmund-Thomson syndrome. OS may also present de novo or after RT. These tumors have a classic radiologic appearance. In the extremities, the Codman triangle signifies subperiosteal bone formation. This feature is less frequently seen in the head and neck, where the classic "sunburst"

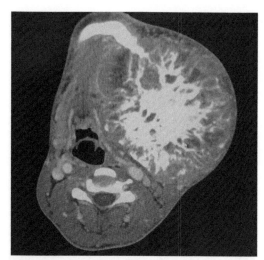

Fig. 1. A destructive mass measuring 11.0 × 11.6 × 12.5 cm in transverse by anteroposterior by craniocaudad dimension involving the left mandibular condyle, coronoid process, ramus, and proximal body with massive sunburst periosteal new bone formation and a large soft-tissue component.

appearance of malignant osteoid formation is observed.

These tumors originate more frequently in the metaphyseal region of extremity long bones, with

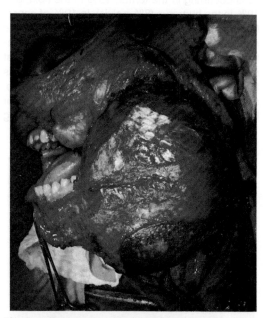

Fig. 2. Intraoperative photo of osteosarcoma. Lower cheek flap is elevated (with the parotid to protect the facial nerve) past the inferior border of the mandible to the level of the zygomatic process.

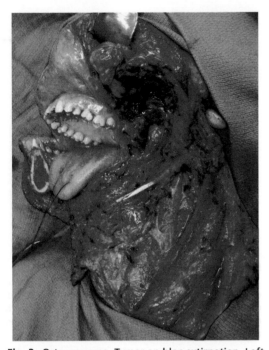

Fig. 3. Osteosarcoma. Tumor en bloc extirpation. Left neck dissection levels I, II, and III (sparing internal jugular, spinal accessory, and sternocleidomastoid muscle), left segmental mandibulectomy, and re-section of floor of mouth. The patient then proceeded to have rectus abdominis myocutaneous flap reconstruction.

42% occurring in the femur, 19% in the tibia, and 10% in the humerus (8% pelvis). In 10% of cases, tumors occur within the head and neck. The mandible, maxilla, and skull are the common locations, with the mandible reported as the most common site. The posterior body of the ramus is the classic mandibular location. The alveolar ridge, sinus floor, and palate are classic maxillary tumor locations. As such, the common presenting

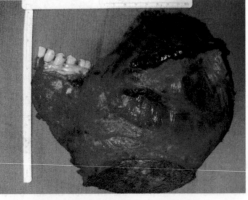

Fig. 4. Osteosarcoma. Operative specimen.

features of these tumors include dental pain and loose teeth, or a painless mass.

There is no formal consensus on what constitutes "best" treatment for adult OS. Surgery, radiation, and chemotherapy have been used singularly or in combination. Neoadjuvant therapy allows for the evaluation of the response to chemotherapy and can be an effective prognostic tool that helps in the selection of optimal adjuvant therapy. Osteosarcomas metastasize relatively early and there is good evidence that neoadjuvant chemotherapy, surgery, and adjuvant chemotherapy improve disease-free survival and overall survival.[24–26] Several drugs have been used that are active in the treatment of OS, including high-dose methotrexate with leucovorin rescue, adriamycin, cisplatin, ifosfamide, and cyclophosphamide. These drugs are administered in various combinations in an effort to destroy pulmonary micrometastases, which are considered to be present in at least 80% of extremity OS patients at the time of diagnosis.[27] Head and neck OS have a reduced likelihood of distant metastases, with only 7% to 17% of patients developing distant disease, most commonly to the brain or lung.[28,29]

A 3-fold improvement in disease-free survival was realized in the 1980s with the introduction of neoadjuvant chemotherapy in the treatment of extremity osteosarcoma in the pediatric population. The variants, especially dedifferentiated parosteal osteosarcoma and dedifferentiated well-differentiated intraosseous osteosarcoma, are more common in adults than in children, which may account, in part, for inferior prognosis in adults. Can we extrapolate the advantages of neoadjuvant chemotherapy, in particular in the pediatric population, to adults? There are several conflicting studies.[30,31] The Memorial Sloan Kettering Cancer Center (MSKCC) experience for head and neck OS could not demonstrate improved local control, decreased distant metastases, or improved disease-specific survival with the addition of neoadjuvant chemotherapy to conventional management.[32] Furthermore, the response to neoadjuvant chemotherapy is difficult to interpret clinically or radiologically because the bony architecture of the tumor does not allow the mass to "shrink," even if there is significant tumor necrosis. MSKCC reports 3-year overall, disease-specific, and recurrence-free survival rates of approximately 81%, 81%, and 73%, respectively.[32]

What is clear is that complete surgical excision to achieve negative surgical margins, especially of the involved bone, is crucial to local control, as well as recurrence-free and disease-specific survival. A positive margin carries with it a significant drop in survival from 75% to 35%.[28,33] It would seem reasonable to administer neoadjuvant chemotherapy to patients with high-grade OS or lesions when initial resection is likely to incur the risk of positive surgical margins or a poor functional result. Routine node dissection is not required, given the low rates of cervical nodal metastases. Occasionally removal of neck nodes may facilitate removal of the tumor or be required if there is extension into the soft tissues of the neck. M.D. Anderson indicated that radiation (at doses of 55–60 Gy) improved local control, disease-specific survival, and overall survival for patients with OS of the head and neck with a positive or uncertain resection margin after surgery.[23]

ANGIOSARCOMA

Angiosarcomas represent one of the most challenging sarcomas in head and neck cancer. These lesions are malignant endothelial cell tumors of lymphatic or vascular origin, found primarily in elderly patients (85% of patients >60 years[34]), with men affected twice as frequently as women. There is no agreed treatment consensus, with scattered phase 2 and no phase 3 trials reported in the literature. Angiosarcomas, which are most commonly characterized by immunohistochemical staining for CD31, may arise in any soft tissue or viscera, and cutaneous angiosarcomas typically involve the scalp. Several risk factors exist for the development of angiosarcoma, including radiation-induced (typically 5–10 years postradiation[35]); chronic lymphedema; Milroy syndrome; exogenous toxins including vinyl chloride, arsenic, and anabolic steroids; and familial syndromes including BRCA 1, BRCA 2, Nf-I, Maffucci syndrome, and Klippel-Trenaunay syndrome.[36] Angiosarcomas can be divided into multiple subcategories, including primary cutaneous angiosarcoma, radiation-associated angiosarcoma, primary breast angiosarcoma, and soft-tissue angiosarcoma. A microarray analysis of 222 angiosarcoma specimens describes high levels of expression of VEGF-A, VEGF-C, KIT, phospho-AKT, phospho-4eBP1, and eIF4E, with significant correlative associations between KIT and p-AKT, as well as p-AKT and VEGF-A, VEGF-C, p-4eBP1, and eIF4E.[37]

Angiosarcoma has two clinical presentations in the head and neck. The first is a nodular strawberry-like lesion and the second is an ecchymotic diffuse lesion presenting most commonly on the scalp. Between 20% and 45% of patients have distant metastases on presentation.[38,39] The main prognostic indicators are size (>5 cm), high grade, and anatomic site (scalp) of presentation.[40–43]

Angiosarcoma is such a rare entity that it requires an individual therapeutic approach for each patient. Surgery and adjuvant RT are most commonly quoted treatment strategies; however, diffuse tumor margins often inhibit satisfactory oncologic excision and hence the necessity for an adjunctive and potentially neoadjuvant therapy.[40,43,44] What type of surgery should be performed on these often elderly patients? Given the poor survival statistics that accompany this diagnosis, an efficient one-step surgical procedure to facilitate negative surgical margins when feasible is desirable. Let us consider the scalp and its extensive vascular network. Various arterial branches from the internal and external carotid, for example, occipital, supratrochlear, and superficial temporal arteries, form anastomoses in the subcutaneous and subgaleal layers. There are also draining venous outlets that follow the arteries, and emissary veins drain to the sagittal sinus of the brain.[45] This elaborate communication system allows for rapid malignant dissemination of angiosarcoma. Tumor extirpation, confirmation of surgical margins, and resurfacing with a split-thickness skin graft is a rapid and reliable technique which, though rarely feasible, allows patients to receive adjunctive therapy in a timely fashion. It must be said that in this disease although a negative margin is gratifying, it does not correlate with survival in several studies.[46,47] RT has been shown to improve survival rates in combination with chemotherapy, with reduced local recurrence. Some investigators even suggest definitive radiation without surgical intervention with or without chemotherapy may offer sufficient primary local control.[41,48,49] The fact that 20% to 45% of patients present with distant metastases emphasizes the importance of effective systemic chemotherapy. However, its role in the literature is debated. Some studies report improved outcomes with the administration of chemotherapeutic agents such as doxorubicin, ifosfamide, cyclophosphamide, dacarbazine, paclitaxel, interferon, and interleukin-2.[39,49,50] Other investigators have not shown improved outcomes with chemotherapy.[44,46,51]

In nonmetastatic angiosarcoma, a personalized treatment approach starting with consultation with multidisciplinary colleagues is appropriate. Combined modality therapies are applied with surgical extirpation with wide 2-cm margins and adjunctive RT of 60 to 66 Gy to wide treatment fields. Neoadjuvant or adjuvant taxane (antiangiogenic activity) therapy is used in selected cases. Angiosarcoma tumors of the scalp and neck have a 10-year relative survival rate of 13.8%, highlighting the challenges that remain in offering meaningful cancer care.[34]

RHABDOMYOSARCOMA

Rhabdomyosarcoma (RMS) is a pediatric sarcoma that rarely occurs in adults (**Figs. 5** and **6**). Using the Surveillance, Epidemiology, and End Results Program, between 1973 and 2007 the incidence of RMS of the head and neck has increased significantly, with an annual percentage change of 1.16%.[52]

RMS in the pediatric age groups has changed, with a dramatic improvement in survival from 25% in the early 1970s to 71% by 2001. This improvement can be attributed to the formation of 3 pediatric cooperative cancer study groups, the Intergroup Rhabdomyosarcoma Study Group (IRSG) in 1972, and the more recent Children's Oncology Group (COG) and COG Soft Tissue Sarcoma (COG-STS). These groups stand as an example of the benefits of academic and clinical cooperation, with survival advantages attributed to improved staging, risk stratification, local therapy, and supportive care.[53]

There are two main pathologic entities, embryonal and alveolar, which are pathologically distinct. In contrast to other sarcomas, the head and neck is the common site where it occurs. Success in management has been largely credited to multiagent chemotherapeutic regimens introduced by IRSG. Early response to therapy by radiologic imaging does not predict long-term failure-free survival (FFS). The difficulty is that CT and MRI modalities are poor at distinguishing residual viable tumor from necrotic tumor or scar tissue. The role of PET scanning is actively being investigated in terms of both tumor response to therapy and the role in detecting metastatic disease in bone and lymphatics.[54,55]

Intergroup Rhabdomyosarcoma Study IV (IRS-IV) emphasized that therapy for children with RMS should be risk directed and based primarily

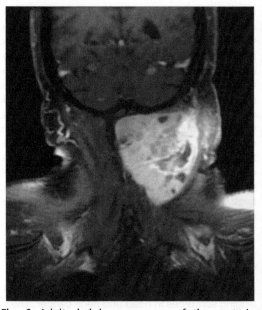

Fig. 6. Adult rhabdomyosarcoma of the posterior neck musculature in a 70-year-old man.

on tumor site, histology, and extent of disease.[56] IRS-V used the concept of risk stratification to conduct studies based on clinical and biological prognostic factors. Risk stratification is based on pretreatment staging and a surgical and pathologic clinical grouping established by IRSG.[57,58]

The clinical group is based on the extent of residual tumor after surgery (when possible) with consideration of regional lymph node involvement. The IRS staging system is based on tumor size, invasiveness, nodal status, and site of primary tumor. Two other prognostic factors are tumor histology and age at diagnosis. Clinical grouping and staging are highly predictive of outcome.

Three-year FFS rates for patients on IRS-IV were 83% for group I, 86% for group II, and 73% for group III. Patients with group IV (metastatic) RMS have long-term FFS rates of less than 30%. For IRS-IV, 3-year FFS rates were 86% for stage 1, 80% for stage 2, and 68% for stage 3.[56,59,60]

Pediatric patients younger than 10 years more commonly present with embryonal RMS (ERMS). In patients older than 10 years, alveolar RMS (ARMS) is the most common diagnosis. Age is also an independent prognostic factor in IRS-III and IRS-IV. Infants have a worse outcome because of increased local failure.[61] In infants and adolescents survival is decreased, owing to the higher frequency of undifferentiated or alveolar histiotypes.

The results from IRS-III and IRS-IV facilitate the placement of patients within low, intermediate, and high risk stratifications. Patients with clinical

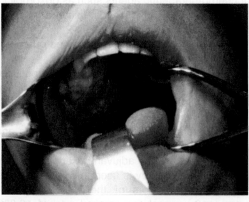

Fig. 5. Alveolar rhabdomyosarcoma of the hard palate in a 22-year-old man after chemoradiation, requiring salvage surgery.

and biological features that place them in a low risk stratification have a 3-year FFS of 88%, and include 2 subsets of patients. Low-risk subset 1 is stage 1, group I/IIA; stage 2, group I; and stage 1, group III (orbit only) ERMS. Low-risk subset 2 is stage I, group IIB/IIC, or group III (nonorbit).

Nonmetastatic ERMS (stage 2, 3, group 3) are considered to have intermediate-risk RMS and have a 5-year FFS of 73%. In addition, patients with ARMS (stage 1–3, groups I–III), with a 5-year FFS of 65%, are included in the intermediate-risk category. Patients younger than 10 years with metastatic disease were also included within the intermediate category. High-risk stage 4, group IV RMS (ERMS >10 years of age and ARMS of any age) have an estimated FFS of less than 20%.[53]

The more recent COG studies apply varying chemotherapeutic combinations to assess response using the risk-stratified patient populations.[62,63] The many drugs that have been used include vincristine, dactinomycin, doxorubicin, ifosfamide, etoposide, cyclophosphamide, actinomycin-D, topotecan, irinotecan, cixutumumab, and temozolomide.

Outcomes in adult patients with rhabdomyosarcoma are poor, with a 5-year survival rate of approximately 30%. In adolescents and adults there is a greater predilection for alveolar and pleomorphic (malignant fibrous histiocytoma morphologic similarities) histopathologic subtypes and anatomic presentation within truncal or extremity sites. Females may have a treatment and overall survival advantage.[64] One of the questions still unanswered is, can we extrapolate the results and experience of the pediatric populations to adults? This point of conjecture will be a subject of debate at ASCO 2012, and further studies are awaited for clarification.

Another area of RMS that is gaining momentum is the gene status of the tumor. Unlike other pediatric embryonal tumors such as neuroblastoma and medulloblastoma, the current risk stratification does not formally use any molecular or genetic data. The genetic characteristics may eventually be included within the risk stratification, along with clinical features. The PAX3/FOXO1 fusion gene was discovered in 1993.[65] The PAX3/FOXO1 fusion gene, resulting from the stable reciprocal translocation of chromosomes 2 and 13, is a signature genetic change found only in ARMS, and is thought to be in part responsible for its malignant phenotype. The presence of PAX3/7-FOXO1 translocation in adult patients is significantly associated with a higher frequency of metastatic disease. There are reports that PAX3-FOXO1 exerts pleiotropic effects, including increasing cell proliferation, promoting cell survival, suppressing terminal differentiation, promoting invasive characteristics, and supporting angiogenesis.[66] Positivity of this gene may have a negative prognostic impact; however, how to incorporate this within the current stratifications is challenging. A recent study reported the PAX3/FOXO1 fusion gene status can be combined with just 2 other variables (ie, IRS TNM stage and age at diagnosis) to make an effective prognostic risk classifier.[67]

LIPOSARCOMA

Liposarcomas account for 35% to 45% of all soft-tissue sarcomas.[68] Approximately 2% of liposarcomas present within the head and neck region, and as such there is a limited reporting of these tumors in the literature. The remaining liposarcomas are reported within the extremities and retroperitoneum.[69] There is a male predominance, and etiologic factors include Nf-1 gene, trauma, and irradiation. There are several subtypes that include well-differentiated, myxoid, pleomorphic, and round cell tumors. Well-differentiated and myxoid are considered low grade, whereas pleomorphic and round cell are high-grade tumors. Survival is determined by subtype of tumor, grade, size, and anatomic site of presentation.

In a study of 76 patients the principal determinant of outcome was histologic grade. Five-year survival was 100% for well-differentiated, 73% for myxoid, 42% for pleomorphic, and 0% for round cell liposarcomas.[69]

Disease-specific survival in a study of 30 patients reported 100% for well-differentiated and myxoid variants, 60% for round cell, and 45% for pleomorphic liposarcomas.[68] The difficulty with these tumors is local recurrence. In particular, in the head and neck a compartmental resection, which is possible in the extremities, is restricted by vital neurovascular structures. Thus postoperative RT is frequently undergone. Radiation improves local recurrence; however, it may not have any impact on overall survival. Local recurrence can be reduced from 60% to 40% with the addition of radiation.[70] In 1954 a study of 105 patients reported improved 5-year survival of 88% for surgery plus radiotherapy, versus 67% for surgery alone. More recently a study of 76 patients from the Royal Marsden in London reported a 5-year survival rate of 83% for surgery and radiotherapy versus 63% for radiotherapy alone.[69] In 7 trials from Europe (with a total of 2185 patients) with advanced liposarcomas, adjuvant radiation had a significantly higher control rate of 36% compared with other soft-tissue sarcomas.[71]

It is agreed that surgery with negative margins is the gold-standard treatment for all histologic subtypes of liposarcomas. Adjuvant radiotherapy is used for high-grade tumors, large tumors and positive margins. Round cell and pleomorphic tumors may metastasize to the lungs, and a yearly chest radiograph is advised.

FIBROSARCOMA

Fibrosarcomas and MFHs share common histopathologic similarities. Fibrosarcomas present in the fourth and fifth decades and most commonly present with a painless mass. Radiation exposure is again a well-documented etiologic factor, with 10% of patients having prior radiation exposure.[72]

A study of 29 patients in 1991 reported an absolute 5-year survival of 62%. Tumor grade was the most important prognostic factor, followed by tumor size and surgical margin status identified in the study.[73] A study of 132 cases reported the cumulative probability of distant metastases was 34% at 1 year, 52% at 2 years, and 63% at 5 years. Distant metastases occurred as late as 22 years after surgery, and metastasis was not significantly associated with surgical margin.[74]

Patients with low-grade lesions and adequate surgical margins are sufficiently treated with surgery alone. Patients with high-grade lesions or positive surgical margins should receive adjuvant RT. Fibrosarcomas have an improved prognosis compared with other sarcomas, with 5-year survival of up to 82%.[2]

CHONDROSARCOMA

Chondrosarcomas are rare tumors (**Fig. 7**). The gross appearance of these tumors is similar to that of other benign chondroid tumors; a smooth, grayish-white hue with a pedunculated and/or friable granular appearance. Myxoid and mesenchymal chondrosarcoma subtypes constitute a substantial portion of head and neck cases. The myxoid variant is an extraskeletal tumor arising in soft tissues and most commonly in the extremities.[75] Mesenchymal chondrosarcomas are recognized as aggressive tumors, as they have a tendency to be high grade. Immunohistochemical and cytogenic studies have identified features similar to those of Ewing sarcoma. Low-grade chondrosarcomas may be difficult to discriminate, from a histopathologic perspective, from osteochondroma, enchondroma, or synovial chondromatosis. Conversely, high-grade tumors may also have histopathologic similarities to tumors such as chondroblastic osteosarcoma, fibrosarcoma, or malignant fibrous histiocytoma.

The National Cancer Database Report of chondrosarcomas in 2000 noted that owing to the rarity

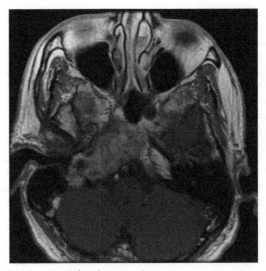

Fig. 7. T1-weighted magnetic resonance postcontrast images of a chondrosarcoma demonstrating enhancement, ruling out other pathology such as a cholesteatoma. The classic paramedian position is noted.

of this disease, it was not possible to accrue a sufficiently large patient population to statistically analyze the impact of proton ocular RT on survival.[76] The anecdotal benefit of RT has long been recognized; however, there are no randomized or nonrandomized prospective studies to suggest where and when RT should be used. Traditionally RT was reserved for inoperable recurrence or inadequate surgical margins. In 1984 Harwood and colleagues[77] reported that chondrosarcomas may indeed be radioresponsive after a long-standing belief that these tumors were radioresistant. This proposal was explained by observations that these tumors had an extracellular matrix, low percentage of dividing cells, and limited vascularity.[78] Further anecdotal reports emerged of an adjunctive response in advanced disease, cases of positive margins, or surgically unresectable tumors.[79,80] Chondrosarcomas are still considered relatively radioresistant tumors and require greater than 65 Gy. Conventional external beam RT with photons has considerable morbidity, especially for lesions at the skull base. Proton beam therapy, on the other hand, has been used to deliver high-energy doses to the tumor while minimizing scatter to adjacent critical anatomic structures; this relates to a minimal exit dose after energy deposition in the target volume.[81] Furthermore, proton therapy has a small but appreciably greater biological effective dose. The first article of the benefits of proton therapy reported 3 cases of skull-base chondrosarcomas treated with surgery and postoperative proton beam therapy mixed with photons. Local control rates at 5 years of up to 85% to 100% have been reported with mixed photon-proton and proton-only protocols.[82–84]

Intensity-modulated RT (IMRT) allows for the delivery of high-dose conformal photons using either standard fractionation, as with protons, or hypofractionated regimens. No data regarding outcomes for skull-base chondrosarcomas exist, but IMRT allows for the delivery of doses within the range that can control skull-base chondrosarcomas. With regard to other adjuvant treatments for chondrosarcoma, there are no definitive reports in the literature supporting the role of adjunctive chemotherapy in the management of these tumors despite the theoretical advantage of chemotherapy in patients with high-grade tumors, with a high risk of distant dissemination.[85] Similarly, there is no palliative benefit reported in the literature. In the absence of proven tumoricidal effect for chondrosarcomas, chemotherapy has no current role in management. In terms of management of the neck, the authors do not recommend elective neck dissections in clinically and radiographically negative necks. The literature also rarely reports regional or distant metastatic disease at presentation.[86,87]

SUMMARY

Soft-tissue sarcomas are a diverse group of mesenchymal tumors with distinct prognostic implications. These tumors present relatively rarely in the head and neck region, with the exception of pediatric rhabdomyosarcoma. Surgery remains the main therapeutic option with the exception of rhabdomyosarcoma, Ewing sarcoma, and angiosarcoma, for which chemoradiation or neoadjuvant chemotherapy is the preferred first-line treatment. Positive margins, large tumors, and high-grade histology continue to have an impact on local control and overall survival.

The sarcoma story is far from complete, and improved histopathologic classification and combined modality therapy are necessary for translation to improved overall survival in both adult and pediatric patients.

REFERENCES

1. Brockstein B. Management of sarcomas of the head and neck. Curr Oncol Rep 2004;6(4):321–7.
2. Sturgis EM, Potter BO. Sarcomas of the head and neck region. Curr Opin Oncol 2003;15(3):239–52.
3. Willers H, Hug EB, Spiro IJ, et al. Adult soft tissue sarcomas of the head and neck treated by radiation and surgery or radiation alone: patterns of failure and prognostic factors. Int J Radiat Oncol Biol Phys 1995;33(3):585–93.
4. Roh JL, Moon BJ, Kim JS, et al. Use of ^{18}F-fluorodeoxyglucose positron emission tomography in patients with rare head and neck cancers. Clin Exp Otorhinolaryngol 2008;1(2):103–9.
5. Kresnik E, Mikosch P, Gallowitsch HJ, et al. Evaluation of head and neck cancer with ^{18}F-FDG PET: a comparison with conventional methods. Eur J Nucl Med 2001;28(7):816–21.
6. Roh JL, Ryu CH, Choi SH, et al. Clinical utility of ^{18}F-FDG PET for patients with salivary gland malignancies. J Nucl Med 2007;48(2):240–6.
7. Schuetze SM, Patel S. Should patients with high-risk soft tissue sarcoma receive adjuvant chemotherapy? Oncologist 2009;14(10):1003–12.
8. Chen SA, Morris CG, Amdur RJ, et al. Adult head and neck soft tissue sarcomas. Am J Clin Oncol 2005;28(3):259–63.
9. O'Brien JE, Stout AP. Malignant fibrous xanthomas. Cancer 1964;17:1445–55.
10. Zagars GK, Ballo MT, Pisters PW, et al. Prognostic factors for patients with localized soft-tissue sarcoma treated with conservation surgery and radiation therapy: an analysis of 1225 patients. Cancer 2003;97(10):2530–43.
11. Weiss SW, Enzinger FM. Malignant fibrous histiocytoma: an analysis of 200 cases. Cancer 1978; 41(6):2250–66.
12. Enzinger FM. Malignant fibrous histiocytoma 20 years after Stout. Am J Surg Pathol 1986;10(Suppl 1):43–53.
13. Patel SG, See AC, Williamson PA, et al. Radiation induced sarcoma of the head and neck. Head Neck 1999;21(4):346–54.
14. Bilici S, Yigit O, Taskin U, et al. Recurrence of a simultaneous tumor of the parotid gland and scalp skin malignant fibrous histiocytoma. J Craniofac Surg 2011;22(5):1898–999.
15. Satomi T, Watanabe M, Kaneko T, et al. Radiation-induced malignant fibrous histiocytoma of the maxilla. Odontology 2011;99(2):203–8.
16. Patel SR. Radiation-induced sarcoma. Curr Treat Options Oncol 2000;1(3):258–61.
17. Davidson T, Westbury G, Harmer CL. Radiation-induced soft-tissue sarcoma. Br J Surg 1986;73(4): 308–9.
18. Sheppard DG, Libshitz HI. Post-radiation sarcomas: a review of the clinical and imaging features in 63 cases. Clin Radiol 2001;56(1):22–9.
19. Wiklund TA, Blomqvist CP, Raty J, et al. Postirradiation sarcoma. Analysis of a nationwide cancer registry material. Cancer 1991;68(3):524–31.
20. Clark DW, Moore BA, Patel SR, et al. Malignant fibrous histiocytoma of the head and neck region. Head Neck 2011;33(3):303–8.
21. Oda Y, Tamiya S, Oshiro Y, et al. Reassessment and clinicopathological prognostic factors of malignant

fibrous histiocytoma of soft parts. Pathol Int 2002; 52(9):595–606.

22. Fernandes R, Nikitakis NG, Pazoki A, et al. Osteogenic sarcoma of the jaw: a 10-year experience. J Oral Maxillofac Surg 2007;65(7):1286–91.

23. Guadagnolo BA, Zagars GK, Raymond AK, et al. Osteosarcoma of the jaw/craniofacial region: outcomes after multimodality treatment. Cancer 2009;115(14):3262–70.

24. Benjamin RS, Patel SR. Pediatric and adult osteosarcoma: comparisons and contrasts in presentation and therapy. Cancer Treat Res 2009;152:355–63.

25. Eilber F, Giuliano A, Eckardt J, et al. Adjuvant chemotherapy for osteosarcoma: a randomized prospective trial. J Clin Oncol 1987;5(1):21–6.

26. Link MP, Goorin AM, Miser AW, et al. The effect of adjuvant chemotherapy on relapse-free survival in patients with osteosarcoma of the extremity. N Engl J Med 1986;314(25):1600–6.

27. Jaffe N. Osteosarcoma: review of the past, impact on the future. The American experience. Cancer Treat Res 2009;152:239–62.

28. Ha PK, Eisele DW, Frassica FJ, et al. Osteosarcoma of the head and neck: a review of the Johns Hopkins experience. Laryngoscope 1999;109(6):964–9.

29. Mark RJ, Sercarz JA, Tran L, et al. Osteogenic sarcoma of the head and neck. The UCLA experience. Arch Otolaryngol Head Neck Surg 1991; 117(7):761–6.

30. Smeele LE, Kostense PJ, van der Waal I, et al. Effect of chemotherapy on survival of craniofacial osteosarcoma: a systematic review of 201 patients. J Clin Oncol 1997;15(1):363–7.

31. Kassir RR, Rassekh CH, Kinsella JB, et al. Osteosarcoma of the head and neck: meta-analysis of nonrandomized studies. Laryngoscope 1997;107(1): 56–61.

32. Patel SG, Meyers P, Huvos AG, et al. Improved outcomes in patients with osteogenic sarcoma of the head and neck. Cancer 2002;95(7):1495–503.

33. Daw NC, Mahmoud HH, Meyer WH, et al. Bone sarcomas of the head and neck in children: the St Jude Children's Research Hospital experience. Cancer 2000;88(9):2172–80.

34. Albores-Saavedra J, Schwartz AM, Henson DE, et al. Cutaneous angiosarcoma. Analysis of 434 cases from the surveillance, epidemiology, and end results program, 1973-2007. Ann Diagn Pathol 2011;15(2):93–7.

35. Huang J, Mackillop WJ. Increased risk of soft tissue sarcoma after radiotherapy in women with breast carcinoma. Cancer 2001;92(1):172–80.

36. Young RJ, Brown NJ, Reed MW, et al. Angiosarcoma. Lancet Oncol 2010;11(10):983–91.

37. Lahat G, Dhuka AR, Hallevi H, et al. Angiosarcoma: clinical and molecular insights. Ann Surg 2010; 251(6):1098–106.

38. Abraham JA, Hornicek FJ, Kaufman AM, et al. Treatment and outcome of 82 patients with angiosarcoma. Ann Surg Oncol 2007;14(6):1953–67.

39. Naka N, Ohsawa M, Tomita Y, et al. Angiosarcoma in Japan. A review of 99 cases. Cancer 1995;75(4): 989–96.

40. Ward JR, Feigenberg SJ, Mendenhall NP, et al. Radiation therapy for angiosarcoma. Head Neck 2003; 25(10):873–8.

41. Holden CA, Spittle MF, Jones EW. Angiosarcoma of the face and scalp, prognosis and treatment. Cancer 1987;59(5):1046–57.

42. Aust MR, Olsen KD, Lewis JE, et al. Angiosarcomas of the head and neck: clinical and pathologic characteristics. Ann Otol Rhinol Laryngol 1997;106(11): 943–51.

43. Kohler HF, Neves RI, Brechtbuhl ER, et al. Cutaneous angiosarcoma of the head and neck: report of 23 cases from a single institution. Otolaryngol Head Neck Surg 2008;139(4):519–24.

44. Mark RJ, Poen JC, Tran LM, et al. Angiosarcoma. A report of 67 patients and a review of the literature. Cancer 1996;77(11):2400–6.

45. Buschmann A, Lehnhardt M, Toman N, et al. Surgical treatment of angiosarcoma of the scalp: less is more. Ann Plast Surg 2008;61(4):399–403.

46. Guadagnolo BA, Zagars GK, Araujo D, et al. Outcomes after definitive treatment for cutaneous angiosarcoma of the face and scalp. Head Neck 2011;33(5):661–7.

47. Pawlik TM, Paulino AF, McGinn CJ, et al. Cutaneous angiosarcoma of the scalp: a multidisciplinary approach. Cancer 2003;98(8):1716–26.

48. Sasaki R, Soejima T, Kishi K, et al. Angiosarcoma treated with radiotherapy: impact of tumor type and size on outcome. Int J Radiat Oncol Biol Phys 2002;52(4):1032–40.

49. Ohguri T, Imada H, Nomoto S, et al. Angiosarcoma of the scalp treated with curative radiotherapy plus recombinant interleukin-2 immunotherapy. Int J Radiat Oncol Biol Phys 2005;61(5):1446–53.

50. Skubitz KM, Haddad PA. Paclitaxel and pegylated-liposomal doxorubicin are both active in angiosarcoma. Cancer 2005;104(2):361–6.

51. Adjuvant chemotherapy for localised resectable soft-tissue sarcoma of adults: meta-analysis of individual data. Sarcoma Meta-analysis Collaboration. Lancet 1997;350(9092):1647–54.

52. Turner JH, Richmon JD. Head and neck rhabdomyosarcoma: a critical analysis of population-based incidence and survival data. Otolaryngol Head Neck Surg 2011;145(6):967–73.

53. Malempati S, Hawkins DS. Rhabdomyosarcoma: review of the Children's Oncology Group (COG) Soft-Tissue Sarcoma Committee experience and rationale for current COG studies. Pediatr Blood Canc 2012;59(1):5–10.

54. Burke M, Anderson JR, Kao SC, et al. Assessment of response to induction therapy and its influence on 5-year failure-free survival in group III rhabdomyosarcoma: the Intergroup Rhabdomyosarcoma Study-IV experience—a report from the Soft Tissue Sarcoma Committee of the Children's Oncology Group. J Clin Oncol 2007;25(31):4909–13.

55. Volker T, Denecke T, Steffen I, et al. Positron emission tomography for staging of pediatric sarcoma patients: results of a prospective multicenter trial. J Clin Oncol 2007;25(34):5435–41.

56. Crist WM, Anderson JR, Meza JL, et al. Intergroup rhabdomyosarcoma study—IV: results for patients with nonmetastatic disease. J Clin Oncol 2001; 19(12):3091–102.

57. Maurer HM, Beltangady M, Gehan EA, et al. The intergroup rhabdomyosarcoma study—I. A final report. Cancer 1988;61(2):209–20.

58. Lawrence W Jr, Anderson JR, Gehan EA, et al. Pretreatment TNM staging of childhood rhabdomyosarcoma: a report of the Intergroup Rhabdomyosarcoma Study Group. Children's Cancer Study Group. Pediatric Oncology Group. Cancer 1997;80(6):1165–70.

59. Breneman JC, Lyden E, Pappo AS, et al. Prognostic factors and clinical outcomes in children and adolescents with metastatic rhabdomyosarcoma—a report from the Intergroup Rhabdomyosarcoma Study IV. J Clin Oncol 2003;21(1):78–84.

60. Oberlin O, Rey A, Lyden E, et al. Prognostic factors in metastatic rhabdomyosarcomas: results of a pooled analysis from United States and European cooperative groups. J Clin Oncol 2008;26(14):2384–9.

61. Ferrari A, Casanova M, Bisogno G, et al. Rhabdomyosarcoma in infants younger than one year old: a report from the Italian Cooperative Group. Cancer 2003;97(10):2597–604.

62. Raney RB, Walterhouse DO, Meza JL, et al. Results of the Intergroup Rhabdomyosarcoma Study Group D9602 protocol, using vincristine and dactinomycin with or without cyclophosphamide and radiation therapy, for newly diagnosed patients with low-risk embryonal rhabdomyosarcoma: a report from the Soft Tissue Sarcoma Committee of the Children's Oncology Group. J Clin Oncol 2011;29(10):1312–8.

63. Lager JJ, Lyden ER, Anderson JR, et al. Pooled analysis of phase II window studies in children with contemporary high-risk metastatic rhabdomyosarcoma: a report from the Soft Tissue Sarcoma Committee of the Children's Oncology Group. J Clin Oncol 2006;24(21):3415–22.

64. Esnaola NF, Rubin BP, Baldini EH, et al. Response to chemotherapy and predictors of survival in adult rhabdomyosarcoma. Ann Surg 2001;234(2):215–23.

65. Galili N, Davis RJ, Fredericks WJ, et al. Fusion of a fork head domain gene to PAX3 in the solid tumour alveolar rhabdomyosarcoma. Nat Genet 1993;5(3):230–5.

66. Linardic CM. PAX3-FOXO1 fusion gene in rhabdomyosarcoma. Cancer Lett 2008;270(1):10–8.

67. Missiaglia E, Williamson D, Chisholm J, et al. PAX3/FOXO1 fusion gene status is the key prognostic molecular marker in rhabdomyosarcoma and significantly improves current risk stratification. J Clin Oncol 2012;30(14):1670–7.

68. Davis EC, Ballo MT, Luna MA, et al. Liposarcoma of the head and neck: The University of Texas M. D. Anderson Cancer Center experience. Head Neck 2009;31(1):28–36.

69. Golledge J, Fisher C, Rhys-Evans PH. Head and neck liposarcoma. Cancer 1995;76(6):1051–8.

70. Eeles RA, Fisher C, A'Hern RP, et al. Head and neck sarcomas: prognostic factors and implications for treatment. Br J Cancer 1993;68(1):201–7.

71. Van Glabbeke M, van Oosterom AT, Oosterhuis JW, et al. Prognostic factors for the outcome of chemotherapy in advanced soft tissue sarcoma: an analysis of 2,185 patients treated with anthracycline-containing first-line regimens–a European Organization for Research and Treatment of Cancer Soft Tissue and Bone Sarcoma Group Study. J Clin Oncol 1999;17(1):150–7.

72. Frankenthaler R, Ayala AG, Hartwick RW, et al. Fibrosarcoma of the head and neck. Laryngoscope 1990;100(8):799–802.

73. Mark RJ, Sercarz JA, Tran L, et al. Fibrosarcoma of the head and neck. The UCLA experience. Arch Otolaryngol Head Neck Surg 1991;117(4):396–401.

74. Scott SM, Reiman HM, Pritchard DJ, et al. Soft tissue fibrosarcoma. A clinicopathologic study of 132 cases. Cancer 1989;64(4):925–31.

75. Abramovici LC, Steiner GC, Bonar F. Myxoid chondrosarcoma of soft tissue and bone: a retrospective study of 11 cases. Hum Pathol 1995;26(11): 1215–20.

76. Koch BB, Karnell LH, Hoffman HT, et al. National cancer database report on chondrosarcoma of the head and neck. Head Neck 2000;22(4):408–25.

77. Harwood AR, Cummings BJ, Fitzpatrick PJ. Radiotherapy for unusual tumors of the head and neck. J Otolaryngol 1984;13(6):391–4.

78. Gelderblom H, Hogendoorn PC, Dijkstra SD, et al. The clinical approach towards chondrosarcoma. Oncologist 2008;13(3):320–9.

79. McNaney D, Lindberg RD, Ayala AG, et al. Fifteen year radiotherapy experience with chondrosarcoma of bone. Int J Radiat Oncol Biol Phys 1982;8(2): 187–90.

80. Krochak R, Harwood AR, Cummings BJ, et al. Results of radical radiation for chondrosarcoma of bone. Radiother Oncol 1983;1(2):109–15.

81. Amichetti M, Amelio D, Cianchetti M, et al. A systematic review of proton therapy in the treatment of chondrosarcoma of the skull base. Neurosurg Rev 2010;33(2):155–65.

82. Noel G, Habrand JL, Jauffret E, et al. Radiation therapy for chordoma and chondrosarcoma of the skull base and the cervical spine. Prognostic factors and patterns of failure. Strahlenther Onkol 2003; 179(4):241–8.

83. Noel G, Feuvret L, Ferrand R, et al. Radiotherapeutic factors in the management of cervical-basal chordomas and chondrosarcomas. Neurosurgery 2004; 55(6):1252–60 [discussion: 1260–2].

84. Rosenberg AE, Nielsen GP, Keel SB, et al. Chondrosarcoma of the base of the skull: a clinicopathologic study of 200 cases with emphasis on its distinction from chordoma. Am J Surg Pathol 1999;23(11):1370–8.

85. Bertoni F, Picci P, Bacchini P, et al. Mesenchymal chondrosarcoma of bone and soft tissues. Cancer 1983;52(3):533–41.

86. Finn DG, Goepfert H, Batsakis JG. Chondrosarcoma of the head and neck. Laryngoscope 1984;94(12 Pt 1): 1539–44.

87. Burkey BB, Hoffman HT, Baker SR, et al. Chondrosarcoma of the head and neck. Laryngoscope 1990;100(12):1301–5.

Skull Base Chordomas
Clinical Features, Prognostic Factors, and Therapeutics

Arman Jahangiri, BS[a,b], Brian Jian, MD, PhD[a,b,1],
Liane Miller, BS[a,b,1], Ivan H. El-Sayed, MD[b,c],
Manish K. Aghi, MD, PhD[a,b,d],*

KEYWORDS

• Chordoma • Skull base • Clivus • Radiation therapy • Radiosurgery

KEY POINTS

By the end of this article, physicians should be able to

- Easily identify the clinical presentation as well as the radiologic findings witnessed in patients with skull base chordomas.
- Identify the most appropriate surgical approach based on the location of the skull base chordoma and the advantages and disadvantages associated with each surgical technique.
- Have a better understanding for the role of radiation therapy in the postoperative adjuvant management of chordomas.
- Develop an understanding for some of the current chemotherapies used to treat refractory chordoma and the direction in which future research in chordoma chemotherapy is headed.

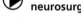 Video of 'Endoscopic endonasal resection of a chordoma' accompanies this article at http://www. neurosurgery.theclinics.com/

INTRODUCTION

Primary bone tumors are uncommon in the skull base. When they do occur, they are typically aggressive even if histologically benign, and most are chondrosarcoma or chordoma. The phenotypes of chondrosarcoma and chordoma may reflect the embryologic development of the skull base because persistent rests of fetal cartilage typically located more laterally and the notochord located medially are believed to give rise to chondrosarcoma and chordoma, respectively, with the former located more laterally and the latter located more medially.

Chordomas, the focus of this review, are rare tumors that arise from the remnant of undifferentiated notochord tissue residing within the vertebral bodies and extra-axial skeleton.[1] Accounting for greater than half of primary tumors of the sacrum, chordomas were originally believed to be found more commonly in the sacrum than the skull base; however, recent evidence suggests an

Disclaimer: AJ is a Howard Hughes Medical Institute Advanced Research Fellow.
[a] Department of Neurological Surgery, University of California, San Francisco, CA 94143, USA; [b] Department of Neurological Surgery at UCSF, Center for Minimally Invasive Skull Base Surgery, University of California San Francisco, CA 94143, USA; [c] Department of Otolaryngology - Head and Neck Surgery, University of California, San Francisco, CA 94115, USA; [d] University of California at San Francisco (UCSF), 505 Parnassus Avenue, Room M779, San Francisco, CA 94143-0112, USA
[1] B Jian and L Miller are contributed equally to work.
* Corresponding author. The University of California at San Francisco (UCSF), 505 Parnassus Avenue, Room M779, San Francisco, CA 94143-0112.
E-mail address: AghiM@neurosurg.ucsf.edu

Neurosurg Clin N Am 24 (2013) 79–88
http://dx.doi.org/10.1016/j.nec.2012.08.007

even distribution amongst the sacrum, mobile spine, and the skull base.[2,3] Of all intracranial tumors, skull base chordomas account for only 0.1% to 0.2%. Skull base chordomas are challenging to manage surgically because of their proximity to the brainstem and other vital neurovascular structures, in addition to an aggressive and locally invasive cellular characteristic.[4,5] Within the skull base, chordomas most often arise extradurally in the clivus, with frequent tendency for intradural invasion; although rare, primary intradural lesions have been reported.[6–9] Although chordomas are considered to be histologically low-grade malignancies,[10] they carry a poor prognosis even after surgery and radiation therapy.[11] This article discusses the pathogenesis, diagnosis, and clinical management of skull base chordomas and presents newly discovered biomarkers, prognostic factors, and benefits of novel chemotherapeutics for this rare aggressive intracranial tumor.

EPIDEMIOLOGY

Chordomas are rare, accounting for only 0.1% to 0.2% of all skull base tumors.[12–14] Analysis of the SEER (Surveillance Epidemiology and End Results) database indicates that chordomas have an overall incidence of 0.08 per 100,000, with peaking incidence between 50 and 60 years of age with a 2:1 male/female ratio.[3,15] They have a low incidence in patients younger than 40 years and are extremely rare in children and adolescents, with these younger patients making up less than 5% of all chordoma cases.[3,16] Chordomas occur in 3 locations (skull base, mobile spine, and sacrum), and evidence suggests an approximately equal distribution (32%, 32.8%, and 29.2% of reported cases, respectively).[3] Chordomas have a poor prognosis because of their insidious nature when an en bloc excision cannot be performed. If untreated, estimated patient survival is 6 to 24 months.[17] However, if treated, median survival is 6 to 8 years, with a 5-year survival rate of 67% to 87%.[3,18,19] In the largest single series to date of patients treated over 25 years, the 5-year and 10-year survival rates are 55% and 36%.[20] Because these tumors are prone to seeding during surgery, it is believed that an en bloc resection is necessary to achieve cure. Patients with lesions of the thoracolumbar spine and appendicular musculoskeletal system have increased survival when an en bloc resection with wide margins is achieved.[21] En bloc resection of lesions involving the C2 vertebra has been reported in only 6 cases, with only 1 of these including the C1 vertbra.[22] Higher lesions involving the clivus are resected in a piecemeal fashion because of the complex anatomy of the surrounding brainstem, cranial nerves (CNs), basilar, vertebral, and carotid arteries.

HISTOPATHOLOGY

Chordomas grossly appear as encapsulated lobular lesions that infiltrate surrounding bone and tissue and can be gray-white to reddish in color.[23] Histologically, they show 3 variants: classic, chondroid, and dedifferentiated.[24] Classic chordoma tumor cells show a lobular arrangement, with intervening fibrous septa. The cells are large, with round nuclei and vacuolated or bubble-containing cytoplasm, often described as physaliferous.[23] Alternatively, chondroid chordomas show features of both chordomas and chondrosarcomas, with chordoma foci surrounded by an extensive cartilaginous matrix.[25] Chordomas were historically identified pathologically based on their physaliferous features and positive immunohistochemical staining for S-100, epithelial membrane antigen, and cytokeratins, but distinction between chondroid chordoma and chondrosarcoma was suboptimal and challenging.[10,26,27] Recently, a nuclear transcription factor, brachyury, was identified as a distinguishing biomarker for chordomas, and in combination with cytokeratin staining, has a sensitivity and specificity greater than 90% for diagnosing chordoma.[28,29]

NEURORADIOLOGIC FINDINGS

Magnetic resonance imaging (MRI) is the main diagnostic modality for skull base chordomas, with chordomas characteristically appearing isointense or hypointense on T1-weighted MRI images and hyperintense on T2-weighted images.[30] Gadolinium enhancement has also been shown but can be variable.[31] Intradural extension can be difficult to predict on preoperative MRI (**Fig. 1**). On computed tomography (CT) scan, chordomas appear as expansive, lytic lesions with bone destruction and soft tissue mass, with varying degrees of enhancement compared with surrounding brain tissue.[32] In addition, on [18F]fluorodeoxyglucose (FDG) positron emission tomography/CT imaging, chordomas show a large, destructive mass with heterogeneous increased uptake of FDG, indicating hypermetabolism.[33]

CLINICAL PRESENTATION

Because of their slow-growing nature, chordomas are often asymptomatic until the late stages of disease, when compression of vital structures may lead to neurologic deficits and pain secondary to mass effect. It is reported that the most common

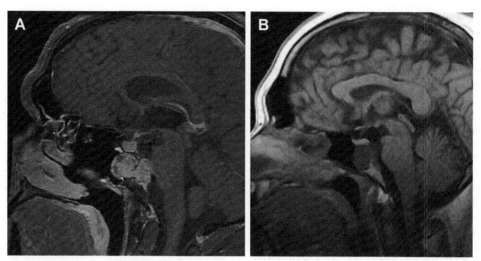

Fig. 1. MRI of chordoma. Preoperative sagittal images of (*A*) a chordoma that showed intradural invasion at surgery, and (*B*) a chordoma that proved to be entirely extradural at surgery.

physical findings at the primary clinical evaluation include in order: sixth nerve palsy, visual field deficits, decreased visual acuity, extraocular motility disorders, and lower CN palsy.[7,14,23,34–36] Dividing the clivus into an upper, mid, and lower section allows for the correlation of tumor location to the ensuing CN deficits. Clival chordomas within the lower clivus present with lower nerve palsies (CN IX, X, XII), whereas tumors in the midclivus often result in diplopia (CNVI) (the most common finding), and chordomas in the upper clivus present with visual acuity deterioration (CNII) and CNIII palsy.[8,23,37–39] Endocrinologic deficits can also occur if chordomas invade superiorly into the sella, but this is rare.[40] Also reported in the literature, but in rare instances, are skull base chordomas presenting with epistaxis and intracranial hemorrhage.[41,42] Although nonspecific, headaches are also common complaints as a result of direct invasion of the dura, compression of trigeminal nerves, diplopia, or increased intracranial pressure.[43]

MANAGEMENT

The therapeutic approach to managing skull base chordomas entails an aggressive surgical procedure with attempts at gross total resection (GTR), followed by focal radiation therapy.[8,44–46]

Surgical Approaches to the Skull Base

Several different approaches have been well documented in the literature for skull base chordomas.[47,48] When a GTR or en bloc resection is not practical, as is often the case for lesions of the clivus, a near total intralesional resection is recommended. Remnant lesions that are small have

been shown to respond well to high-dose radiation therapy, as shown by Potluri and colleagues[49] in a series of 19 patients receiving stereotactic radiosurgery after subtotal resection (STR), with effective control of the small residual tumor volume. Recently, the endoscopic endonasal approach has become increasingly used for clival chordomas. When there is extensive involvement of local neurovascular structures, the operative approach should not be aggressive, and use of radiotherapy and observation of residual tumor should be taken into account, because a patient's quality of life and neurologic function must be of priority when evaluating surgical outcomes.[50,51] The following sections describe 4 of the most common transcranial approaches as well as the endoscopic endonasal approach, which are used solely or in combination with one another for resection of skull base chordomas. Each technique is summarized briefly with a discussion of its benefits and shortcomings. Furthermore, the minimally invasive endonasal endoscopic approach is contrasted with the more invasive cranial procedures, with a focus on the future direction for treatment and neurosurgical approach to the skull base chordoma.

Frontotemporal transcavernous approach

This technique uses an orbitozygomatic osteomy and clinoidal resection to allow the surgeon to reach skull base chordomas invading into the cavernous sinus (CS) and grants exceptional intradural access.[52] This approach is beneficial in that it decreases the amount of brain retraction required for sufficient exposure.[53] Structures such as the supraorbital nerves and vessels, the frontotemporal branch of CNVII, the optic nerve,

CNIII as well as CNIV are at risk for injury with this approach during the resection of clinoid.[43]

Extended frontal transbasal approach

The transbasal approach was first described by Derome,[54] and its use has been modified by the removal of the central segment of the supraorbital bar to become the extended transbasal approach, in which lesions that have superior and inferior extensions can be resected with minimal brain retraction. Midline tumors of the lower to upper clivus that extend into the occipital condyles, foramen magnum, medial CS, or the sphenoethmodial region can be accessed with this approach.[55] This approach fails to gain direct access to the dorsum sella, and chordomas with widespread lateral elements are unreachable. The lateral limits for this approach are CNXII, CNVI, the carotid arteries, and the optic nerve, which places these structures at high risk for operative injury.[43] By further removing the entire supraorbital bar (extensive frontal transbasal approach), one can gain better exposure, specifically for visualization of the contralateral clivus.[56]

Subtemporal and subtemporal-infratemporal approach

The subtemporal approach can be used for gaining access to the posterior CS, upper clivus, middle fossa, petrous apex, and horizontal petrous internal carotid artery. For additional exposure, the subtemporal-infratemporal approach is used, which further aids in visualization of the CS, the clivus all the way to the foramen magnum, the ethmoid, maxillary, and sphenoid sinuses, the orbit, parapharyngeal and retropharyngeal spaces, infratemporal fossa, as well as the orbit.[43] This extensive approach is reserved for instances in which there is involvement of the petroclival bone inferior to the level of the horizontal segment of the petrous internal carotid artery.[57] The most frequent complications of this approach include associated meningitis and cerebrospinal fluid (CSF) leak. Because of the extensive nature of this approach, all CNs are exposed and are put at great risk for injury, whereas the internal carotid artery may be injured during drilling.[43]

Extreme lateral transcondylar approach

Chordomas involving the ventral upper cervical spine, occipital condyles, foramen magnum, and lower clivus can be accessed with this approach.[58] For chordomas located extradurally, the complete transcondylar approach is most often used, but must be conducted in combination with an occipitocervical fusion to guarantee occipitocervical junction stability. Vascular injury to vertebral arteries can lead to cerebellar or brainstem infarction, and lower CN dysfunction and CSF leak are other common complications with this approach.[43]

Endoscopic endonasal approach

The endoscopic endonasal approach is a minimally invasive approach to the clivus as well as the anterior brainstem, serving as the most direct path to the clival chordoma, and has been described in detail by many groups (Video 1).[56,59–61] Reviewing the combined 66 cases published of skull base chordomas undergoing the endoscopic endonasal approach, Fraser and colleagues[56] found the combined GTR rate to be 55%, with a near total resection of more than 95% of the tumor achieved in 7 of 8 patients in their follow-up case series. Other studies have also suggested that this approach to resection of chordomas is equally successful compared with open approaches at achieving total resection.[39,56,61,62] CSF fluid leak occurred in 17% of the patients in the review analysis of Fraser and colleagues.[56] This potential complication is often avoided with the use of the vascularized nasoseptal flap.[63–65] Although all CNs are at risk of injury during this approach, CNVI is at an increased risk because it exits the Dorello canal, coursing toward the CS, a complication for which the risk can be reduced by opening the dura at or below the location of the vertebrobasilar junction identified by neuronavigation. The internal carotid arteries may also be injured during drilling. A contraindication to this approach is when the tumor extends to the lateral edge of the optic nerve, when a different approach should be taken into consideration.[65] For lesions that involve the clivus and extend inferiorly into the upper spine, a combined endonasal endo-oral approach can be performed to limit the need for a palate split or more invasive transoral approach.[66]

POSTOPERATIVE COMPLICATIONS, SURVIVAL, AND RECURRENCE

Postoperative Complications

The Karnofsky performance status (KPS) can be used to assess preoperative and postoperative functional disabilities, and is an appropriate tool for surgeons to determine whether the patient has worsened as a result of surgical treatment, and also an aid to monitor for recurrence, or residual tumor regrowth.[23] In a series of 60 patients, Gay and colleagues[8] found 40% of their patients to show permanent postoperative functional deterioration of about 10 points using the KPS scoring system. A reduction of greater than 10 points was a sign of disease progression as reported by Sen and colleagues,[67] and every patient with this score died as a result of disease progression. In 1 study,[35] GTR was achieved in more than 40% of patients undergoing their first operation, with an overall mortality of only about 5%, a fifth of which were attributed to CSF leaks. The same study reported the risk for CSF leaks to be nearly tripled at 51% for patients undergoing reoperation. Other surgical complications include new CN deficits, nasal speech, and dysphonia, as well as meningitis, all of which are reported to be less common than CSF leaks.[8,35,68,69]

Survival

Chordomas are fatal in many patients, although some patients become long-term survivors, particularly after GTR and appropriate use of adjuvant therapy. A recent study reports their overall 5-year survival rate to be 75%.[38] A review of all cranial chordomas from 1973 to 1995 using the SEER database found relative survival of skull base chordomas to be 65% and 47%, respectively, for 5-year and 10-year survival.[3] Furthermore, the literature[6,23,35,38] reports that when GTR of a tumor is accomplished, the 5-year overall survival increases to 80% or more. Repeat surgery has been shown to correlate with worsened overall survival compared with patients who receive only a single surgery for tumor resection, and the general consensus in the literature is that the best prognosis is achieved via the greatest extent of surgical resection of tumor during the initial operation.[20,35,38]

Recurrence

The literature emphasizes extent of tumor resection as the variable that best correlates with lowering the risk for skull base chordoma recurrence.[70] The progression-free survival (PFS) rate from several studies at 5 years after GTR ranges from 55% to 84%, whereas the corresponding range for patients with a partial or STR is between 36% and 64%.[8,23,35,38,67,71]

RADIATION

Radiation plays a crucial role in the management of chordomas and can be used as an excellent tool for controlling tumor growth.[68,72,73] Chordomas do not generally respond to conventional radiotherapy and their radiosensitivity is limited to high doses, usually in the 70-Gy to 80-Gy dose range.[70] Because skull base chordomas are often located near critical structures such as the optic apparatus, cervical spinal cord, and the brainstem, exposure to high doses of radiation must be limited to prevent permanent damage.[74,75] As a result of these challenges, radiation must be delivered to chordomas in a high dose but focal fashion. The most common radiation modalities used in chordoma management include photon-based radiosurgery methods like Cyber Knife and Gamma Knife and proton beam radiation.[6,69,72,76–78] Proton beam radiation therapy is useful because of its ability to deliver higher doses of radiation to the tumor mass and spare critical nearby structures.[76,79] In a systematic review of 47 articles, Amichetti and colleagues[45] reviewed the data of skull base chordomas treated with proton therapy, and compared it with other irradiation techniques (conventional radiation therapy, ion therapy, radiation therapy, fractionated stereotactic radiation therapy, and radiosurgery). This study showed that the use of protons results in better outcomes compared with the use of conventional photon irradiation, resulting in superior 10-year outcomes.[45] Although the role of proton therapy in patients with residual tumors is well established because it has achieved superior disease control and extended survival, the impact of this treatment has yet to be defined for patients who have undergone GTR after the primary operation.[38] Furthermore, there are only a few centers that offer proton beam therapy, limiting access of many patients to this treatment modality. The likelihood of treatment success is increased for both proton therapy as well as photon-based radiosurgery when the tumor has a smaller volume and is located further from the optic apparatus as well as the brain stem.[68,80] Some of the major complications associated as a result of radiation therapy are pituitary insufficiency (13.2%) as well as involvement of the optic apparatus (4.4%), as described by Austin-Seymour and colleagues[81] in their experience with fractionated proton radiation therapy for chordomas.

CHEMOTHERAPY

Systemic review of the literature[82,83] has found chordoma to be unresponsive to conventional chemotherapies, once again adding to the challenge of managing these tumors. Recent molecular analysis of chordomas has shown an overexpression of several factors that could be targeted by chemotherapy. The tyrosine kinases KIT and BCR-ABL as well as platelet-derived growth factor receptor A (PDGFRA), and PDGFRB are found to be overexpressed in some patients with chordoma, all of which are inhibited via imatinib mesylate (IM), a chemotherapy that inhibits receptor tyrosine kinases.[70] In particular, patients with skull base chordomas are found to have increased expression of PDGFRB, which is likely the primary antitumor target for IM.[84,85] Sunitinib is yet another tyrosine kinase inhibitor that has shown efficacy against chordomas. In a multi-center phase II trial of sunitinib, George and colleagues[86] found that 44% of their patients with chordoma showed stable disease at 16 weeks when treated with sunitinib.

The epidermal growth factor receptor (EGFR) is another marker that has received investigational attention as a possible therapeutic target in chordomas. To determine the EGFR expression of chordomas, Shalaby and colleagues[87] characterized chordomas of 160 patients and found 60% of cases to show EGFR mutations. Using the chordoma cell line U-CH1, as well as patient chordomas from different locations, EGFR overactivation in several chordomas was shown via phosphoreceptor tyrosine kinase array membranes. Tyrphostin, an EGFR inhibitor, showed substantial inhibition of proliferation in the chordoma cell line U-CH1 in vitro and decreased the phosphorylation of EGFR in a manner that was dose-dependent. This study showed that chordomas have abnormal EGFR signaling and suggested that molecular analysis of the EGFR activation status of tumors could be used to select patients who are good candidates for treatment using EGFR antagonists. Furthermore, a case report by Singhal and colleagues[88] reported treatment response with erlotinib, an EGFR tyrosine kinase inhibitor, in a patient unresponsive to a vascular disrupting agent and IM. Other agents shown to be effective in the setting of disease progression after IM treatment include sirolimus and cisplatin.[89,90]

In addition to PDGFR and EGFR, chordomas express receptors and signaling molecules to which currently available molecular-targeted therapies exist, such as c-Met (hepatocyte growth factor receptor) and downstream effectors Phosphatidylinositol 3-kinases (PI3K)/Protein Kinase B (AKT) and mammalian target of rapamycin (mTOR).[84,85,91–97] Therapies targeting several of these molecules have already shown initial success in patients with chordoma and in in vitro models, and combinational therapy is being explored.[89,98,99]

PROGNOSTIC FACTORS AND NOVEL BIOMARKERS

Many factors have been examined and subsequently implicated in the prognosis of chordomas, including extent of surgical resection, previous treatments, and adjuvant therapies.[23] However, many studies have conflicting results. It was initially believed that a younger age at diagnosis was prognostic of a poorer outcome, because previous studies have pointed to the aggressive behavior of chordomas in children, highlighting the hypercellularity, pleomorphism, and high levels of mitotic activity seen in this age group.[100] Moreover, Borda and colleagues[101] reported that the prognosis is worse in these younger patients because of the extremely diverse and malignant pathologic appearance of these tumors observed in children and adolescents. However, more recent studies have indicated that the recurrence rate is lower in patients younger than 40 years and points to a better prognosis.[7,46] Other factors believed to influence prognosis include the classic and chondroid histology (better prognosis compared with dedifferentiated variant), the presence of necrosis and mitotic figures (poor prognosis), metastases (poor prognosis), larger tumor volume at diagnosis (prognostic factor for tumor recurrence and poor prognosis), and Ki67-positive staining (poor prognosis).[5,7,102]

Additional molecular expression marker studies have identified MIB-I, p53, and cyclin D1 as potential predictors of recurrence and prognosis, citing that the proliferative potential of chordomas may be correlated with the combination of p53 overexpression, anaplasia, and high-grade atypia.[103,104]

SUMMARY

Skull base chordomas are exceptionally rare tumors that grow in the clivus, often presenting with CN palsies, headache, and visual field cuts. The management of these tumors entails surgical resection as well as radiation treatment, although many different treatment preferences are presented in the literature. Both extent of resection as well as adjuvant therapy have been shown to affect PFS as well as overall survival. Nonetheless, there is a wide range of variability within the literature of skull base chordomas treated with similar therapeutic options, which may point to a spectrum of heterogeneity amongst these tumors going beyond the extent of resection and radiation therapy. Biomarker profiling has identified several factors that are upregulated in chordomas as prognostic factors, although this literature is by no means complete. The future of skull base chordoma management lies in the increasing recognition of the need for these cases to be referred to surgical centers of excellence, followed by judicious use of high-dose focal radiation techniques like proton beam therapy, and expanding our understanding of the molecular markers responsible for the aggressive behavior of these tumors so that chemotherapies targeting these markers can be incorporated into treatment paradigms in a patient-specific manner.

SUPPLEMENTARY DATA

Supplementary data related to this article can be found online at http://dx.doi.org/10.1016/j.nec.2012.08.007.

REFERENCES

1. Horten BC, Montague SR. In vitro characteristics of a sacrococcygeal chordoma maintained in tissue and organ culture systems. Acta Neuropathol 1976;35(1):13–25.

2. Cheng EY, Ozerdemoglu RA, Transfeldt EE, et al. Lumbosacral chordoma. Prognostic factors and treatment. Spine (Phila Pa 1976) 1999;24(16): 1639–45.

3. McMaster ML, Goldstein AM, Bromley CM, et al. Chordoma: incidence and survival patterns in the United States, 1973-1995. Cancer Causes Control 2001;12(1):1–11.

4. Watkins L, Khudados ES, Kaleoglu M, et al. Skull base chordomas: a review of 38 patients, 1958-88. Br J Neurosurg 1993;7(3):241–8.

5. Pallini R, Maira G, Pierconti F, et al. Chordoma of the skull base: predictors of tumor recurrence. J Neurosurg 2003;98(4):812–22.

6. Tzortzidis F, Elahi F, Wright D, et al. Patient outcome at long-term follow-up after aggressive microsurgical resection of cranial base chordomas. Neurosurgery 2006;59(2):230–7 [discussion: 7].

7. Forsyth PA, Cascino TL, Shaw EG, et al. Intracranial chordomas: a clinicopathological and prognostic study of 51 cases. J Neurosurg 1993;78(5):741–7.

8. Gay E, Sekhar LN, Rubinstein E, et al. Chordomas and chondrosarcomas of the cranial base: results and follow-up of 60 patients. Neurosurgery 1995; 36(5):887–96 [discussion: 96–7].

9. Nishigaya K, Kaneko M, Ohashi Y, et al. Intradural retroclival chordoma without bone involvement: no tumor regrowth 5 years after operation. Case report. J Neurosurg 1998;88(4):764–8.

10. Mitchell A, Scheithauer BW, Unni KK, et al. Chordoma and chondroid neoplasms of the spheno-occiput. An immunohistochemical study of 41 cases with prognostic and nosologic implications. Cancer 1993;72(10):2943–9.

11. Eriksson B, Gunterberg B, Kindblom LG. Chordoma. A clinicopathologic and prognostic study of a Swedish national series. Acta Orthop Scand 1981;52(1):49–58.

12. Samii A, Gerganov VM, Herold C, et al. Chordomas of the skull base: surgical management and outcome. J Neurosurg 2007;107(2):319–24.

13. Sekhar LN, Pranatartiharan R, Chanda A, et al. Chordomas and chondrosarcomas of the skull base: results and complications of surgical management. Neurosurg Focus 2001;10(3):E2.

14. al-Mefty O, Borba LA. Skull base chordomas: a management challenge. J Neurosurg 1997; 86(2):182–9.

15. Di Maio S, Temkin N, Ramanathan D, et al. Current comprehensive management of cranial base chordomas: 10-year meta-analysis of observational studies. J Neurosurg 2011;115(6):1094–105.

16. Wold LE, Laws ER Jr. Cranial chordomas in children and young adults. J Neurosurg 1983;59(6): 1043–7.

17. Kamrin RP, Potanos JN, Pool JL. An evaluation of the diagnosis and treatment of chordoma. J Neurol Neurosurg Psychiatry 1964;27:157–65.

18. Bergh P, Kindblom LG, Gunterberg B, et al. Prognostic factors in chordoma of the sacrum and mobile spine: a study of 39 patients. Cancer 2000;88(9):2122–34.

19. Baratti D, Gronchi A, Pennacchioli E, et al. Chordoma: natural history and results in 28 patients treated at a single institution. Ann Surg Oncol 2003;10(3):291–6.

20. Choi D, Melcher R, Harms J, et al. Outcome of 132 operations in 97 patients with chordomas of the craniocervical junction and upper cervical spine. Neurosurgery 2010;66(1):59–65 [discussion: 65].

21. Cloyd JM, Chou D, Deviren V, et al. En bloc resection of primary tumors of the cervical spine: report of two cases and systematic review of the literature. Spine J 2009;9(11):928–35.

22. Chou D, Acosta F Jr, Cloyd JM, et al. Parasagittal osteotomy for en bloc resection of multilevel cervical chordomas. J Neurosurg Spine 2009; 10(5):397–403.

23. Colli BO, Al-Mefty O. Chordomas of the skull base: follow-up review and prognostic factors. Neurosurg Focus 2001;10(3):E1.

24. Chugh R, Tawbi H, Lucas DR, et al. Chordoma: the nonsarcoma primary bone tumor. Oncologist 2007; 12(11):1344–50.

25. Heffelfinger MJ, Dahlin DC, MacCarty CS, et al. Chordomas and cartilaginous tumors at the skull base. Cancer 1973;32(2):410–20.

26. Henderson SR, Guiliano D, Presneau N, et al. A molecular map of mesenchymal tumors. Genome Biol 2005;6(9):R76.

27. Crapanzano JP, Ali SZ, Ginsberg MS, et al. Chordoma: a cytologic study with histologic and radiologic correlation. Cancer 2001;93(1):40–51.

28. Oakley GJ, Fuhrer K, Seethala RR. Brachyury, SOX-9, and podoplanin, new markers in the skull base chordoma vs chondrosarcoma differential: a tissue microarray-based comparative analysis. Mod Pathol 2008;21(12):1461–9.

29. Jambhekar NA, Rekhi B, Thorat K, et al. Revisiting chordoma with brachyury, a "new age" marker: analysis of a validation study on 51 cases. Arch Pathol Lab Med 2010;134(8):1181–7.

30. Erdem E, Angtuaco EC, Van Hemert R, et al. Comprehensive review of intracranial chordoma. Radiographics 2003;23(4):995–1009.

31. Meyers SP, Hirsch WL Jr, Curtin HD, et al. Chordomas of the skull base: MR features. AJNR Am J Neuroradiol 1992;13(6):1627–36.

32. Meyer JE, Oot RF, Lindfors KK. CT appearance of clival chordomas. J Comput Assist Tomogr 1986; 10(1):34–8.

33. Park SA, Kim HS. F-18 FDG PET/CT evaluation of sacrococcygeal chordoma. Clin Nucl Med 2008; 33(12):906–8.

34. Cho YH, Kim JH, Khang SK, et al. Chordomas and chondrosarcomas of the skull base: comparative analysis of clinical results in 30 patients. Neurosurg Rev 2008;31(1):35–43 [discussion: 43].

35. Crockard HA, Steel T, Plowman N, et al. A multidisciplinary team approach to skull base chordomas. J Neurosurg 2001;95(2):175–83.

36. Pamir MN, Ozduman K. Tumor-biology and current treatment of skull-base chordomas. Adv Tech Stand Neurosurg 2008;33:35–129.

37. Crockard A, Macaulay E, Plowman PN. Stereotactic radiosurgery. VI. Posterior displacement of the brainstem facilitates safer high dose radiosurgery for clival chordoma. Br J Neurosurg 1999; 13(1):65–70.

38. Sen C, Triana AI, Berglind N, et al. Clival chordomas: clinical management, results, and complications in 71 patients. J Neurosurg 2010;113(5): 1059–71.

39. Stippler M, Gardner PA, Snyderman CH, et al. Endoscopic endonasal approach for clival chordomas. Neurosurgery 2009;64(2):268–77 [discussion: 77–8].

40. Stark AM, Mehdorn HM. Images in clinical medicine. Chondroid clival chordoma. N Engl J Med 2003;349(10):e10.

41. Kitai R, Yoshida K, Kubota T, et al. Clival chordoma manifesting as nasal bleeding. A case report. Neuroradiology 2005;47(5):368–71.

42. Levi AD, Kucharczyk W, Lang AP, et al. Clival chordoma presenting with acute brain stem hemorrhage. Can J Neurol Sci 1991;18(4):515–8.

43. Koutourousiou M, Snyderman CH, Fernandez-Miranda J, et al. Skull base chordomas. Otolaryngol Clin North Am 2011;44(5):1155–71.

44. Miller RC, Foote RL, Coffey RJ, et al. The role of stereotactic radiosurgery in the treatment of malignant skull base tumors. Int J Radiat Oncol Biol Phys 1997;39(5):977–81.

45. Amichetti M, Cianchetti M, Amelio D, et al. Proton therapy in chordoma of the base of the skull: a systematic review. Neurosurg Rev 2009;32(4): 403–16.

46. Jian BJ, Bloch OG, Yang I, et al. Adjuvant radiation therapy and chondroid chordoma subtype are associated with a lower tumor recurrence rate of cranial chordoma. J Neurooncol 2010;98(1):101–8.

47. Holzmann D, Reisch R, Krayenbuhl N, et al. The transnasal transclival approach for clivus chordoma. Minim Invasive Neurosurg 2010;53(5–6):211–7.

48. Singh H, Harrop J, Schiffmacher P, et al. Ventral surgical approaches to craniovertebral junction chordomas. Neurosurgery 2010;66(Suppl 3): 96–103.

49. Potluri S, Jefferies SJ, Jena R, et al. Residual postoperative tumour volume predicts outcome after high-dose radiotherapy for chordoma and chondrosarcoma of the skull base and spine. Clin Oncol (R Coll Radiol) 2011;23(3):199–208.

50. Stuer C, Schramm J, Schaller C. Skull base chordomas: management and results. Neurol Med Chir (Tokyo) 2006;46(3):118–24 [discussion: 124–5].

51. Walcott BP, Nahed BV, Mohyeldin A, et al. Chordoma: current concepts, management, and future directions. Lancet Oncol 2012;13(2):e69–76.

52. Hakuba A, Tanaka K, Suzuki T, et al. A combined orbitozygomatic infratemporal epidural and subdural approach for lesions involving the entire cavernous sinus. J Neurosurg 1989;71(5 Pt 1):699–704.

53. Day JD. Surgical approaches to suprasellar and parasellar tumors. Neurosurg Clin North Am 2003; 14(1):109–22.

54. Derome P. Transbasal approach to tumors invading the skull base. In: Schmidek HH, Sweet WH, editors. Operative neurosurgical techniques, indications, methods, and results. Philadelphia: WB Saunders; 1995. p. 427–42.

55. Sekhar LN, Nanda A, Sen CN, et al. The extended frontal approach to tumors of the anterior, middle, and posterior skull base. J Neurosurg 1992;76(2): 198–206.

56. Fraser JF, Nyquist GG, Moore N, et al. Endoscopic endonasal transclival resection of chordomas: operative technique, clinical outcome, and review of the literature. J Neurosurg 2010;112(5):1061–9.

57. Cass SP, Sekhar LN, Pomeranz S, et al. Excision of petroclival tumors by a total petrosectomy approach. Am J Otol 1994;15(4):474–84.

58. Sen CN, Sekhar LN. An extreme lateral approach to intradural lesions of the cervical spine and foramen magnum. Neurosurgery 1990;27(2):197–204.

59. Cavallo LM, Messina A, Cappabianca P, et al. Endoscopic endonasal surgery of the midline skull base: anatomical study and clinical considerations. Neurosurg Focus 2005;19(1):E2.

60. DeMonte F, Diaz E Jr, Callender D, et al. Transmandibular, circumglossal, retropharyngeal approach for chordomas of the clivus and upper cervical spine. Technical note. Neurosurg Focus 2001; 10(3):E10.

61. Frank G, Sciarretta V, Calbucci F, et al. The endoscopic transnasal transsphenoidal approach for

the treatment of cranial base chordomas and chondrosarcomas. Neurosurgery 2006;59(1 Suppl 1): ONS50–7 [discussion: ONS-7].

62. Jho HD, Ha HG. Endoscopic endonasal skull base surgery: Part 3–the clivus and posterior fossa. Minim Invasive Neurosurg 2004;47(1):16–23.

63. Hadad G, Bassagasteguy L, Carrau RL, et al. A novel reconstructive technique after endoscopic expanded endonasal approaches: vascular pedicle nasoseptal flap. Laryngoscope 2006;116(10): 1882–6.

64. Kassam AB, Thomas A, Carrau RL, et al. Endoscopic reconstruction of the cranial base using a pedicled nasoseptal flap. Neurosurgery 2008; 63(1 Suppl 1):ONS44–52 [discussion: ONS-3].

65. Snyderman CH, Pant H, Carrau RL, et al. What are the limits of endoscopic sinus surgery?: the expanded endonasal approach to the skull base. Keio J Med 2009;58(3):152–60.

66. El-Sayed IH, Wu JC, Ames CP, et al. Combined transnasal and transoral endoscopic approaches to the craniovertebral junction. J Craniovertebr Junction Spine 2010;1(1):44–8.

67. Sen C, Triana A. Cranial chordomas: results of radical excision. Neurosurg Focus 2001;10(3):E3.

68. Hug EB, Loredo LN, Slater JD, et al. Proton radiation therapy for chordomas and chondrosarcomas of the skull base. J Neurosurg 1999;91(3):432–9.

69. O'Connell JX, Renard LG, Liebsch NJ, et al. Base of skull chordoma. A correlative study of histologic and clinical features of 62 cases. Cancer 1994; 74(8):2261–7.

70. Gagliardi F, Boari N, Riva P, et al. Current therapeutic options and novel molecular markers in skull base chordomas. Neurosurg Rev 2012;35(1):1–13 [discussion: 4].

71. Pamir MN, Kilic T, Ture U, et al. Multimodality management of 26 skull-base chordomas with 4-year mean follow-up: experience at a single institution. Acta Neurochir (Wien) 2004;146(4):343–54 [discussion: 354].

72. Austin JP, Urie MM, Cardenosa G, et al. Probable causes of recurrence in patients with chordoma and chondrosarcoma of the base of skull and cervical spine. Int J Radiat Oncol Biol Phys 1993; 25(3):439–44.

73. Castro JR, Linstadt DE, Bahary JP, et al. Experience in charged particle irradiation of tumors of the skull base: 1977–1992. Int J Radiat Oncol Biol Phys 1994;29(4):647–55.

74. Tai PT, Craighead P, Bagdon F. Optimization of radiotherapy for patients with cranial chordoma. A review of dose-response ratios for photon techniques. Cancer 1995;75(3):749–56.

75. Mendenhall WM, Mendenhall CM, Lewis SB, et al. Skull base chordoma. Head Neck 2005;27(2): 159–65.

76. Munzenrider JE, Liebsch NJ. Proton therapy for tumors of the skull base. Strahlenther Onkol 1999; 175(Suppl 2):57–63.

77. Muthukumar N, Kondziolka D, Lunsford LD, et al. Stereotactic radiosurgery for chordoma and chondrosarcoma: further experiences. Int J Radiat Oncol Biol Phys 1998;41(2):387–92.

78. Noel G, Feuvret L, Calugaru V, et al. Chordomas of the base of the skull and upper cervical spine. One hundred patients irradiated by a 3D conformal technique combining photon and proton beams. Acta Oncol 2005;44(7):700–8.

79. Suit HD, Goitein M, Munzenrider J, et al. Definitive radiation therapy for chordoma and chondrosarcoma of base of skull and cervical spine. J Neurosurg 1982;56(3):377–85.

80. Debus J, Schulz-Ertner D, Schad L, et al. Stereotactic fractionated radiotherapy for chordomas and chondrosarcomas of the skull base. Int J Radiat Oncol Biol Phys 2000;47(3):591–6.

81. Austin-Seymour M, Munzenrider J, Goitein M, et al. Fractionated proton radiation therapy of chordoma and low-grade chondrosarcoma of the base of the skull. J Neurosurg 1989;70(1):13–7.

82. York JE, Kaczaraj A, Abi-Said D, et al. Sacral chordoma: 40-year experience at a major cancer center. Neurosurgery 1999;44(1):74–9 [discussion: 9–80].

83. Azzarelli A, Quagliuolo V, Cerasoli S, et al. Chordoma: natural history and treatment results in 33 cases. J Surg Oncol 1988;37(3):185–91.

84. Casali PG, Messina A, Stacchiotti S, et al. Imatinib mesylate in chordoma. Cancer 2004;101(9): 2086–97.

85. Orzan F, Terreni MR, Longoni M, et al. Expression study of the target receptor tyrosine kinase of imatinib mesylate in skull base chordomas. Oncol Rep 2007;18(1):249–52.

86. George S, Merriam P, Maki RG, et al. Multicenter phase II trial of sunitinib in the treatment of nongastrointestinal stromal tumor sarcomas. J Clin Oncol 2009;27(19):3154–60.

87. Shalaby A, Presneau N, Ye H, et al. The role of epidermal growth factor receptor in chordoma pathogenesis: a potential therapeutic target. J Pathol 2011;223(3):336–46.

88. Singhal N, Kotasek D, Parnis FX. Response to erlotinib in a patient with treatment refractory chordoma. Anticancer Drugs 2009;20(10):953–5.

89. Stacchiotti S, Marrari A, Tamborini E, et al. Response to imatinib plus sirolimus in advanced chordoma. Ann Oncol 2009;20(11):1886–94.

90. Casali PG, Stacchiotti S, Grosso F, et al. Adding cisplatin (CDDP) to imatinib (IM) re-establishes tumor response following secondary resistance to IM in advanced chordoma. 2007 ASCO Annual Meeting Proceedings Part I; 2007: 10038. 2007.

91. Tamborini E, Miselli F, Negri T, et al. Molecular and biochemical analyses of platelet-derived growth factor receptor (PDGFR) B, PDGFRA, and KIT receptors in chordomas. Clin Cancer Res 2006;12(23):6920–8.

92. Fasig JH, Dupont WD, LaFleur BJ, et al. Immuno-histochemical analysis of receptor tyrosine kinase signal transduction activity in chordoma. Neuropathol Appl Neurobiol 2008;34(1):95–104.

93. Weinberger PM, Yu Z, Kowalski D, et al. Differential expression of epidermal growth factor receptor, c-Met, and HER2/neu in chordoma compared with 17 other malignancies. Arch Otolaryngol Head Neck Surg 2005;131(8):707–11.

94. Deniz ML, Kilic T, Almaata I, et al. Expression of growth factors and structural proteins in chordomas: basic fibroblast growth factor, transforming growth factor alpha, and fibronectin are correlated with recurrence. Neurosurgery 2002;51(3):753–60 [discussion: 60].

95. Naka T, Kuester D, Boltze C, et al. Expression of hepatocyte growth factor and c-MET in skull base chordoma. Cancer 2008;112(1):104–10.

96. Han S, Polizzano C, Nielsen GP, et al. Aberrant hyperactivation of akt and mammalian target of rapamycin complex 1 signaling in sporadic chordomas. Clin Cancer Res 2009;15(6):1940–6.

97. Presneau N, Shalaby A, Idowu B, et al. Potential therapeutic targets for chordoma: PI3K/AKT/TSC1/TSC2/mTOR pathway. Br J Cancer 2009;100(9):1406–14.

98. Stacchiotti S, Longhi A, Ferraresi V, et al. Phase II study of imatinib in advanced chordoma. J Clin Oncol 2012;30(9):914–20.

99. Hof H, Welzel T, Debus J. Effectiveness of cetuximab/gefitinib in the therapy of a sacral chordoma. Onkologie 2006;29(12):572–4.

100. Coffin CM, Swanson PE, Wick MR, et al. Chordoma in childhood and adolescence. A clinicopathologic analysis of 12 cases. Arch Pathol Lab Med 1993;117(9):927–33.

101. Borba LA, Al-Mefty O, Mrak RE, et al. Cranial chordomas in children and adolescents. J Neurosurg 1996;84(4):584–91.

102. Wu Z, Zhang J, Zhang L, et al. Prognostic factors for long-term outcome of patients with surgical resection of skull base chordomas–106 cases review in one institution. Neurosurg Rev 2010;33(4):451–6.

103. Matsuno A, Sasaki T, Nagashima T, et al. Immuno-histochemical examination of proliferative potentials and the expression of cell cycle-related proteins of intracranial chordomas. Hum Pathol 1997;28(6):714–9.

104. Naka T, Fukuda T, Chuman H, et al. Proliferative activities in conventional chordoma: a clinicopathologic, DNA flow cytometric, and immunohistochemical analysis of 17 specimens with special reference to anaplastic chordoma showing a diffuse proliferation and nuclear atypia. Hum Pathol 1996;27(4):381–8.

Skull Base Chondrosarcoma
Evidence-Based Treatment Paradigms

Orin Bloch, MD, Andrew T. Parsa, MD, PhD*

KEYWORDS

- Chondrosarcoma • Skull base • Microsurgery • Radiotherapy

KEY POINTS

- Cranial chondrosarcomas are generally low-grade, indolent malignancies of bone that cause morbidity through compression of neurovascular structures at the skull base.
- The mainstay of treatment for chondrosarcoma is surgical resection followed by adjuvant radiation therapy. Although proton beam radiotherapy is often considered optimal management, multiple radiotherapy modalities demonstrate equivalent efficacy in long-term studies.
- Surgical approaches should be selected based on pattern of tumor growth and attachment, as well as preexisting neurologic deficits.
- Although chemotherapy is not currently part of the standard treatment regimen for chondrosarcoma, emerging molecular-targeted therapies may contribute to tumor control in the future.

INTRODUCTION

Chondrosarcoma is the second most common primary malignancy of bone, arising from cells of chondroid (cartilage) origin throughout the axial and appendicular skeleton.[1] Only 1% of chondrosarcomas arise in the skull base, and account for 6% of all skull-base tumors.[2] The vast majority of cranial tumors are low to intermediate grade with indolent growth and low metastatic potential.[3] However, their intimate association with critical neural and vascular structures at the skull base often results in significant morbidity from tumor growth and surgical intervention. The mainstay of therapy for chondrosarcoma is surgical resection, with fractionated radiation therapy used to limit recurrence. Recently, radiosurgery has been investigated as an alternative to fractionated radiotherapy. There has been little role for chemotherapy in the treatment of this disease.

This review examines the published literature on the management of cranial chondrosarcoma, including the importance of the extent of microsurgical resection and the multiple modalities of adjuvant radiation including radiosurgery, proton beam, and heavy-particle radiotherapy. The goal is to provide an evidence-based guideline for the management of this rare and complicated disease. In addition, laboratory evidence is presented for new molecular targets to improve emerging chemotherapies for chondrosarcoma.

PATHOLOGY

Cranial chondrosarcoma occurs primarily at the base of the skull, arising from rests of chondrocytes within the synchondroses of the basilar skull bones.[4] Tumors are found most often in the paraclival region arising from sphenopetrosal, petro-occipital, or spheno-occipital synchondroses.[5] The vast majority of lesions involve the bone of the clivus, and extend anteriorly into the parasellar sinuses or middle cranial fossa (30%–50%), or posteriorly into the posterior fossa (50%).[6] Although invasion through the dura is uncommon, compression of the brainstem or temporal lobe is frequent at presentation (**Fig. 1**).[6] Cranial chondrosarcoma occurs preferentially at the skull base,

Disclosure: The authors have no financial interests in the results of this article.
Department of Neurological Surgery, University of California, San Francisco, 505 Parnassus Avenue, M-779, San Francisco, CA 94143-0112, USA
* Corresponding author.
E-mail address: parsaa@neurosurg.ucsf.edu

Neurosurg Clin N Am 24 (2013) 89–96
http://dx.doi.org/10.1016/j.nec.2012.08.002
1042-3680/13/$ – see front matter © 2013 Published by Elsevier Inc.

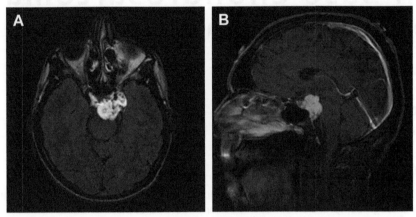

Fig. 1. T2-weighted axial FLAIR (*A*) and T1-weighted contrast enhanced sagittal (*B*) images of a patient with a skull-base chondrosarcoma centered at the left petroclival junction.

owing to differences in bone development between the cranial vault and the basilar structures. The cranial vault grows primarily by intramembranous ossification, whereas the basilar skull bones develop by endochondral ossification and retain rests of chondrocytes into maturity, which can undergo malignant degeneration.[7,8] Most chondrosarcomas develop sporadically, although tumor formation has been associated with diseases of endochondroma formation including Ollier disease and Maffucci syndrome.[9]

Chondrosarcoma manifests grossly as a destructive, mineralized mass that invades bone and extends into soft tissues. Lesions typically grow in bone with an infiltrative pattern, replacing normal marrow elements and spreading through Haversian canals.[10] Eventually lesions break through the cortex and invade surrounding soft tissue. Histopathologically, chondrosarcomas can be of the conventional, mesenchymal, clear-cell, or dedifferentiated type. Almost all skull-base tumors are the conventional type, with rare (<10%) mesenchymal lesions reported.[11] The clear cell and dedifferentiated types do not occur in the axial skeleton. Conventional chondrosarcoma can be composed of hyaline or myxoid cartilage, or a combination of the two (**Fig. 2**). Conventional lesions are graded according to the degree of cellularity, cytologic atypia, and mitotic activity on a 3- or 4-tiered scale, with the lowest grade representing well-differentiated tumors. In the 2 largest case series of skull-base chondrosarcoma reported in the literature, 50% of the lesions were low grade (grade 1) and nearly 90% were low to intermediate grade (grade 1–2).[11,12] High-grade, poorly differentiated lesions of the conventional subtype are rare in all anatomic locations, and identification of aggressively invasive,

poorly differentiated cartilage should raise the possibility of chondroblastic osteosarcoma.

Chondrosarcomas, especially low-grade tumors, have relatively indolent growth compared with other sarcomas. Nonetheless, they are highly invasive and have the potential for distant metastasis. Approximately 7% of patients have distant metastasis, which is most commonly seen with high-grade conventional tumors and the mesenchymal subtype.[11]

CLINICAL PRESENTATION

Data from the national cancer database indicates that the median age at presentation for cranial chondrosarcoma is 51 years, with a slight male predominance (55% of cases).[11] Most cases (85%) occur in non-Hispanic white patients. As indicated previously, most cases demonstrate a conventional histologic subtype with low-grade pathology. Fewer than 10% of cases are of the mesenchymal subtype, and these patients tend

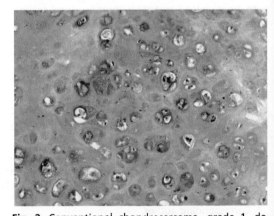

Fig. 2. Conventional chondrosarcoma, grade 1, demonstrating hyaline architecture (hematoxylin and eosin; original magnification ×200).

to be younger, with greater than 60% of cases occurring in patients younger than 30 years.[11]

Because of the location of most tumors in the skull base, along the spheno-petro-clival junction, the majority of patients present with symptoms of cranial nerve compression. In a series of 33 patients with cranial chondrosarcoma managed at the University of California, San Francisco, the most common presenting symptoms were headache and diplopia, with nearly 50% of patients presenting with palsy of the sixth cranial nerve.[13] A similar presentation was reported by groups from the Barrow Neurological Institute and the International Neuroscience Institute in Hannover, whose series contained mostly clivus-invading tumors causing sixth-nerve dysfunction from compression within the Dorello canal.[6,14] By contrast, the group from the House Clinic reported on 8 patients with a predominance of petrous apex tumors extending into the cerebellopontine angle who all presented with dysfunction of the lower cranial nerve.[15] The presence of particular cranial-nerve deficits at presentation can be an important factor in the selection of surgical approach, especially with regard to function of cranial nerve VIII and the feasibility of a transpetrosal approach.

The differential diagnosis for skull-base lesions in the typical location of a cranial chondrosarcoma includes chordoma, other primary bone tumors, skull-base metastases, meningiomas, schwannomas of the lower cranial nerve, neuroblastoma, and lymphoma. Although any of these expansile lesions may cause bony remodeling, erosive destruction of the petrous apex or clivus is not generally associated with lesions other than chondrosarcoma, chordoma, or metastases. Therefore, in addition to magnetic resonance imaging, computed tomography and plain radiographs may be useful in determining the diagnosis.

MANAGEMENT
Surgical Resection

The current standard for initial treatment of cranial chondrosarcoma is surgical resection to obtain a definitive tissue diagnosis and maximally cytoreduce the tumor. Selection of the approach to the skull base is principally determined by the primary direction of tumor growth and the involved cranial nerves.[6] Tumors involving the petrous apex and upper third of the clivus with extension anteriorly into the Meckel cave or the cavernous sinus are often addressed through a frontotemporal orbitozygomatic approach, or a pure middle-fossa craniotomy with subtemporal dissection. By contrast, posteriorly and inferiorly directed tumors extending below the internal acoustic canal are best treated through a retrosigmoid or transpetrosal approach. Large tumors may require a combined petrosal/middle-fossa approach or a staged procedure. Among a group of combined modern surgical case series for skull-base chondrosarcoma, approximately a third of tumors were resected via an anterior approach, a third via a posterolateral approach, and a third via alternative approaches including transfacial and transsphenoidal approaches.[5,6,13,14,16] Endoscopic transnasal approaches have also been reported with success for specific tumors.[17]

Preoperative cranial-nerve deficits are common in cranial chondrosarcoma patients, with the most common presenting symptom being diplopia secondary to dysfunction of cranial nerve VI. Given the invasive nature of chondrosarcoma and the difficult location of most tumors at the skull base, improvements in cranial nerve deficits after surgery are uncommon, and the potential for causing new deficits with surgery is significant. In their series of 18 patients, Samii and colleagues[6] found that 16 of 18 (89%) patients had at least a partial cranial neuropathy at presentation. After surgical resection 25% had new cranial nerve deficits, whereas 55% had no improvement in their preoperative symptoms. Similarly, Sekhar and colleagues[16] reported 41% new cranial neuropathies in their series of 22 chondrosarcoma patients. In addition to cranial neuropathies, modern surgical series also report an approximately 10% to 15% rate of vascular injury, 10% rate of cerebrospinal fluid leak, and up to 5% perioperative mortality.[14,16,18] Given the relatively high morbidity of such procedures, there is some controversy in the literature regarding the goals of operations. Some investigators have argued that the goal for initial intervention should be aggressive gross-total resection, as this offers the possibility for a surgical cure. The groups that advocate this approach report a complete resection achieved in 50% to 60% of patients.[5,6] By contrast, others have argued for an approach using maximal safe cytoreduction followed by radiotherapy to control residual tumor growth. In general, 5-year tumor-recurrence rates and overall survival were 70% to 80% and 80% to 90%, respectively, regardless of the approach used.[6,12,13,18] There is no direct evidence to suggest that extent of resection at the initial operation offers any recurrence or survival benefit when adjuvant radiation is given.

The authors previously performed a systemic analysis of the published literature on cranial chondrosarcoma, disaggregating the data from individual case series to statistically evaluate predictors of tumor recurrence[19] and overall survival.[20] The cumulative data from all published series of cranial chondrosarcoma demonstrates a recurrence-free survival of 78% at 5 years and an overall survival of 88% at 5 years. The greatest predictor of outcome was tumor histology, with mesenchymal-type tumors showing nearly 5-fold greater 5-year mortality (**Fig. 3**A). Within conventional type tumors, tumor grade was associated with worsening survival (**Fig. 3**B). However, mesenchymal and high-grade conventional tumors were rare, representing fewer than 11% of all cases. For the majority of patients, outcome was significantly affected by the use of adjuvant radiation. The authors' analysis found that 5-year mortality was decreased from 25% to 9% with the addition of any form of radiation (**Fig. 3**C). A recent case series of 6 patients with cranial chondrosarcoma treated with surgical resection followed by fractionated radiotherapy found 100% tumor control at 5 years irrespective of the residual tumor volume after resection, which ranged from 0 to 28.7 cm³.[21] Although this is a small series it supports the trend seen in the surgical data, which indicate that survival outcomes are approximately the same regardless of the extent of surgical resection. A robust analysis of the effect of extent of resection on a group of chondrosarcoma patients with equivalent adjuvant therapy has not been performed, leaving this issue open for debate.

Radiation Therapy

The use of adjuvant radiation following surgical resection for cranial chondrosarcoma has been shown to improve tumor control and overall survival in several case series.[12,13,18] As indicated, the authors' systematic analysis demonstrates decreased tumor recurrence and mortality at 5 years with the addition of radiation to surgical resection.[19,20] Radiotherapy for chondrosarcoma may be given by multiple modalities including fractionated photon radiotherapy, particle (proton, carbon ion) radiotherapy, or stereotactic radiosurgery. There are no class I data suggesting that the use of one radiation modality is preferable to any other. Support for the use of each radiation technique is based on individual case series.

Conventional fractionated radiotherapy has been used the longest as an adjuvant to surgical resection for cranial chondrosarcoma. Most case series report delivering a median total dose of 55 to 65 Gy.[18,22] Before the availability of the

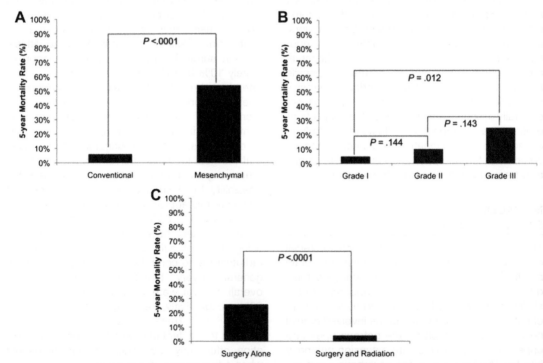

Fig. 3. Effects of tumor histology and treatment on overall survival. (*A*) The effect of histologic subtype on 5-year mortality demonstrates a nearly 5-fold increase in mortality associated with mesenchymal histology. (*B*) The effect of tumor grade on 5-year mortality in conventional type tumors demonstrates increased mortality with increasing tumor grade. (*C*) The effect of adjuvant radiation following surgery compared with surgery alone demonstrates a significant reduction in 5-year mortality with the addition of radiotherapy. (*From* Bloch O, Jian BJ, Yang I, et al. A systematic review of intracranial chondrosarcoma and survival. J Clin Neurosci 2009;16:1547–51; with permission.)

highly conformal techniques used today, such as intensity-modulated radiation therapy (IMRT), these doses were delivered using external beam radiotherapy with quantifiable dose distribution to the brainstem and other critical structures at the skull base. Using photon radiotherapy, most groups report 5-year progression-free survival rates of greater than 80%, and overall survival greater than 90%.[13,18,22] Little early or late radiation toxicity is reported with this technique.

Charged-particle radiotherapy, specifically proton beam therapy, has gained favor for the treatment of skull-base bony malignancies over the last 2 decades. Because of the sharp fall-off in ionizing energy at the target, known as the Bragg peak effect, protons can be used to deliver higher energy with high levels of conformality. In addition, there is a theorized radiobiological advantage to protons in comparison with photons. Proton therapy was first used at the skull base to treat chordomas, which are more radioresistant and have a greater tendency to recur, requiring higher doses of radiation than can safely be administered by conventional photon therapy. This technique has subsequently been applied to the treatment of cranial chondrosarcomas. Case series reporting proton beam as adjuvant therapy for chondrosarcoma administer substantially higher median doses than photon therapy, ranging from 60 to 79 cobalt Gray equivalents (CGE).[23,24] Similar to the results with photon radiotherapy, progression-free survival at 5 years for proton therapy ranges from 75% to 95% and overall survival ranges from 85% to 100%.[12,23–26] Although there are no studies directly comparing the efficacy of proton versus photon therapy, tumor control and overall survival rates reported in individual studies for both techniques are concordant. Studies on proton beam therapy do report a delayed radiation toxicity rate of 4% to 14% for grade 3 and 4 toxicities.[23–26]

In addition to protons, carbon-ion particle therapy has been used for the treatment of skull-base chondrosarcomas. Carbon ions have the same energy characteristics as protons, allowing high doses to be given to conformal fields, with a possible benefit of a greater radiobiological response to the carbon. The Radiation Oncology Group in Heidelberg has published their case series of 54 patients with skull-base chondrosarcomas treated with carbon ions, in which they report a tumor control rate of 89% and overall survival of 98% at 5 years.[27] These investigators treated patients to a median dose of 60 CGE in hypofractionated daily fractions of 3.0 CGE, and reported a delayed radiation toxicity rate of 10% for low-grade (1 and 2) toxicities and 2% for high-grade (3 and 4) toxicities.

An alternative adjuvant to fractionated radiotherapy with photons or protons is radiosurgery. Stereotactic radiosurgery (SRS) can deliver a highly conformal large radiation dose to a tumor in a single session, and has become the standard in radiotherapy for benign skull-base tumors. The use of SRS as adjuvant therapy for malignant skull-base tumors, including chondrosarcoma, has been increasing, with several published reports on outcomes. In 2007, the Pittsburgh group reported their series of 10 patients with skull-base chondrosarcomas who received adjuvant radiation with SRS with a median marginal dose of 16 Gy.[28] The investigators reported a 5-year tumor control rate of 80% and no acute or late radiation toxicity. In 2012, they updated their series of 22 chondrosarcoma patients treated with SRS, including 7 patients treated with SRS as primary therapy without surgery.[29] In the updated series, they reported a median marginal treatment dose of 15 Gy with a 22% rate of radiation toxicity. The tumor control rate and overall survival at 5 years were 70%. Similar tumor control and survival rates have been published by other groups in mixed studies of SRS for chordoma and chondrosarcoma.[30–33] Although no direct comparisons of SRS with fractionated radiotherapy or proton beam therapy have been made in a controlled study, the reported outcomes for SRS as adjuvant or primary therapy for skull-base chondrosarcoma appear to be worse than those reported with other radiation modalities. The poor outcomes may be due, in part, to the mixed nature of the patients treated in the SRS studies, including patients who have had multiple resections and are receiving salvage therapy. Nonetheless, with the data available at this time, it is not possible to claim that SRS provides improved or even equivalent outcomes to fractionated radiotherapy for treatment following initial surgical resection.

Chemotherapy

Chemotherapy for chondrosarcoma in the skull base and throughout the axial skeleton has been largely ineffective and is, therefore, not part of the standard therapy for this tumor. Occasionally chemotherapy has been used as salvage therapy for multiply recurrent or metastatic disease. A review of the national cancer database demonstrated that less than 5% of patients with head and neck chondrosarcoma received any form of chemotherapy, usually in conjunction with surgical resection.[11] There is little evidence beyond individual case reports to suggest efficacy of any chemotherapeutic regimen. This area is one that requires further clinical research.

EMERGING THERAPIES

Although modern therapy for skull-base chondrosarcoma can achieve tumor control rates in excess of 80% at 5 years and overall survival in excess of 90% at 5 years, there remains significant room for improvement in long-term outcomes. Surgical resection is the standard of care for initial therapy, although the goals of therapy have been debated. Surgical morbidity for these tumors is significant, and despite improvements in skull-base surgical techniques, gross-total resection is only achievable in 50% of cases at best. Furthermore, there is no evidence that greater extent of resection improves outcome, as multiple studies have demonstrated equivalent survival regardless of the extent of resection when adjuvant radiation is given. Further improvements in surgical techniques are not likely to substantially improve outcomes for patients with skull-base chondrosarcoma. Radiation therapy, too, has seen substantial improvements in technique over the past 2 decades, but new modalities of radiation have not been shown to clearly improve outcome. With high-energy conformal techniques for photon therapy (IMRT) and particle therapy (proton beam), radiation can be delivered safely with minimal toxicity, but survival has not substantially improved. Further data, including controlled prospective trials of multiple radiation modalities, are necessary to determine the ideal method of adjuvant radiation for chondrosarcoma.

With limitations in the efficacy of surgery and radiation for control of skull-base chondrosarcomas, the future of treatment may be new molecular therapies targeted at chondrosarcoma cell proliferation and invasion. Unfortunately, in vitro and animal models of cranial chondrosarcoma are not readily available. Most of the studies on chondrosarcoma genetics and signaling come from appendicular specimens and cultures. The authors recently reviewed the literature on known signaling

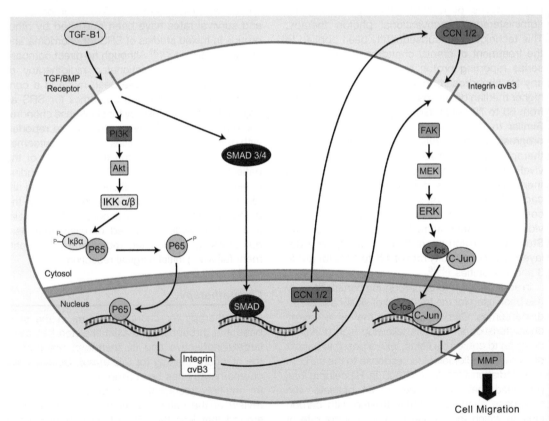

Fig. 4. Proposed interaction of chondrosarcoma with the extracellular environment. Inflammation results in transforming growth factor (TGF) receptor ligand formation, which binds to receptor and activated phosphoinositide 3-kinase (PI3K)/Akt activity and pathogenic upregulation of integrins and their ligands. When integrins bind ligands at the cell surface, the FAK-MEK-ERK pathway is activated, resulting in matrix metalloproteinase (MMP) expression and degradation of the extracellular matrix. BMP, bone morphogenetic protein; IKK, I-κB kinase. (*From* Bloch O, Sughrue ME, Mills SA, et al. Signaling pathways in cranial chondrosarcoma: potential molecular targets for directed chemotherapy. J Clin Neurosci 2011;18:881–5; with permission.)

pathways in chondrosarcoma that have been shown to functionally influence tumor-cell invasion and migration.[34] Chronic inflammation in rests of chondrocytes was found to result in activation of transforming growth factor receptors by inflammatory cytokines in the extracellular matrix of bone and cartilaginous tissue. Activation of these receptors leads to upregulation of integrins, specifically integrin $\alpha_v\beta_3$, through phosphoinositide (PI) 3-kinase signaling. When these integrins bind to constituents of the extracellular matrix at the cell surface, the FAK-MEK-ERK pathway is activated, leading to production of matrix metalloproteinases and degradation of the extracellular matrix, facilitating tumor invasion (**Fig. 4**). Small molecular inhibitors of the PI3-kinase and MEK pathways are currently in early-phase clinical trials as chemotherapeutic agents for other malignancies. This evidence suggests that these inhibitors may have some benefit in preventing tumor growth and invasion in skull-base chondrosarcoma. Further investigation, including coordinated multicentered clinical trials, will be necessary to study new interventions for this rare disease.

SUMMARY

Skull-base chondrosarcomas are indolent but invasive malignant tumors in locations that are often difficult to treat. Based on the available data, standard therapy should consist of maximal safe surgical resection with a goal of cytoreduction, followed by adjuvant fractionated radiotherapy with photons or protons. Further studies are necessary to determine whether one modality of radiotherapy has any advantage over the other. For conventional low-grade tumors, progression-free and overall survival at 5 years is high with this treatment paradigm. Negative predictors of outcome include mesenchymal tumor histology, high tumor grade, or a lack of appropriate adjuvant radiation. Chemotherapy is not currently a part of standard therapy, but new agents targeting specific molecular pathways may prove to be efficacious in the future.

REFERENCES

1. Chow WA. Update on chondrosarcomas. Curr Opin Oncol 2007;19:371–6.
2. Richardson MS. Pathology of skull base tumors. Otolaryngol Clin North Am 2001;34:1025–42, vii.
3. Weber AL, Brown EW, Hug EB, et al. Cartilaginous tumors and chordomas of the cranial base. Otolaryngol Clin North Am 1995;28:453–71.
4. Korten AG, ter Berg HJ, Spincemaille GH, et al. Intracranial chondrosarcoma: review of the literature and report of 15 cases. J Neurol Neurosurg Psychiatry 1998;65:88–92.
5. Tzortzidis F, Elahi F, Wright DC, et al. Patient outcome at long-term follow-up after aggressive microsurgical resection of cranial base chondrosarcomas. Neurosurgery 2006;58:1090–8 [discussion: 8].
6. Samii A, Gerganov V, Herold C, et al. Surgical treatment of skull base chondrosarcomas. Neurosurg Rev 2009;32:67–75 [discussion].
7. Lau DP, Wharton SB, Antoun NM, et al. Chondrosarcoma of the petrous apex. Dilemmas in diagnosis and treatment. J Laryngol Otol 1997;111:368–71.
8. Watters GW, Brookes GB. Chondrosarcoma of the temporal bone. Clin Otolaryngol Allied Sci 1995;20:53–8.
9. Noel G, Feuvret L, Calugaru V, et al. Chondrosarcomas of the base of the skull in Ollier's disease or Maffucci's syndrome—three case reports and review of the literature. Acta Oncol 2004;43:705–10.
10. Rosenberg AE. Pathology of chordoma and chondrosarcoma of the axial skeleton. In: Harsh GR, editor. Chordomas and chondrosarcomas of the skull base and spine. New York: Thieme; 2003. p. 8–15.
11. Koch BB, Karnell LH, Hoffman HT, et al. National cancer database report on chondrosarcoma of the head and neck. Head Neck 2000;22:408–25.
12. Rosenberg AE, Nielsen GP, Keel SB, et al. Chondrosarcoma of the base of the skull: a clinicopathologic study of 200 cases with emphasis on its distinction from chordoma. Am J Surg Pathol 1999;23:1370–8.
13. Oghalai JS, Buxbaum JL, Jackler RK, et al. Skull base chondrosarcoma originating from the petroclival junction. Otol Neurotol 2005;26:1052–60.
14. Wanebo JE, Bristol RE, Porter RR, et al. Management of cranial base chondrosarcomas. Neurosurgery 2006;58:249–55 [discussion: 55].
15. Brackmann DE, Teufert KB. Chondrosarcoma of the skull base: long-term follow-up. Otol Neurotol 2006;27:981–91.
16. Sekhar LN, Pranatartiharan R, Chanda A, et al. Chordomas and chondrosarcomas of the skull base: results and complications of surgical management. Neurosurg Focus 2001;10:E2.
17. Frank G, Sciarretta V, Calbucci F, et al. The endoscopic transnasal transsphenoidal approach for the treatment of cranial base chordomas and chondrosarcomas. Neurosurgery 2006;59:ONS50–7 [discussion: ONS-7].
18. Gay E, Sekhar LN, Rubinstein E, et al. Chordomas and chondrosarcomas of the cranial base: results and follow-up of 60 patients. Neurosurgery 1995;36:887–96 [discussion: 96–7].
19. Bloch OG, Jian BJ, Yang I, et al. Cranial chondrosarcoma and recurrence: a systematic review. Skull Base 2010;20:149–56.

20. Bloch OG, Jian BJ, Yang I, et al. A systematic review of intracranial chondrosarcoma and survival. J Clin Neurosci 2009;16:1547–51.

21. Potluri S, Jefferies SJ, Jena R, et al. Residual postoperative tumour volume predicts outcome after high-dose radiotherapy for chordoma and chondrosarcoma of the skull base and spine. Clin Oncol (R Coll Radiol) 2011;23:199–208.

22. Cho YH, Kim JH, Khang SK, et al. Chordomas and chondrosarcomas of the skull base: comparative analysis of clinical results in 30 patients. Neurosurg Rev 2008;31:35–43 [discussion].

23. Hug EB, Loredo LN, Slater JD, et al. Proton radiation therapy for chordomas and chondrosarcomas of the skull base. J Neurosurg 1999;91:432–9.

24. Noel G, Habrand JL, Mammar H, et al. Combination of photon and proton radiation therapy for chordomas and chondrosarcomas of the skull base: the Centre de Protontherapie D'Orsay experience. Int J Radiat Oncol Biol Phys 2001;51:392–8.

25. Weber DC, Rutz HP, Pedroni ES, et al. Results of spot-scanning proton radiation therapy for chordoma and chondrosarcoma of the skull base: the Paul Scherrer Institut experience. Int J Radiat Oncol Biol Phys 2005;63:401–9.

26. Amichetti M, Amelio D, Cianchetti M, et al. A systematic review of proton therapy in the treatment of chondrosarcoma of the skull base. Neurosurg Rev 2010;33:155–65.

27. Schulz-Ertner D, Nikoghosyan A, Hof H, et al. Carbon ion radiotherapy of skull base chondrosarcomas. Int J Radiat Oncol Biol Phys 2007;67:171–7.

28. Martin JJ, Niranjan A, Kondziolka D, et al. Radiosurgery for chordomas and chondrosarcomas of the skull base. J Neurosurg 2007;107:758–64.

29. Iyer A, Kano H, Kondziolka D, et al. Stereotactic radiosurgery for intracranial chondrosarcoma. J Neurooncol 2012;108:535–42.

30. Hasegawa T, Ishii D, Kida Y, et al. Gamma Knife surgery for skull base chordomas and chondrosarcomas. J Neurosurg 2007;107:752–7.

31. Koga T, Shin M, Saito N. Treatment with high marginal dose is mandatory to achieve long-term control of skull base chordomas and chondrosarcomas by means of stereotactic radiosurgery. J Neurooncol 2010;98:233–8.

32. Krishnan S, Foote RL, Brown PD, et al. Radiosurgery for cranial base chordomas and chondrosarcomas. Neurosurgery 2005;56:777–84 [discussion: 84].

33. Forander P, Rahn T, Kihlstrom L, et al. Combination of microsurgery and Gamma Knife surgery for the treatment of intracranial chondrosarcomas. J Neurosurg 2006;105(Suppl):18–25.

34. Bloch O, Sughrue ME, Mills SA, et al. Signaling pathways in cranial chondrosarcoma: potential molecular targets for directed chemotherapy. J Clin Neurosci 2011;18:881–5.

Temporal Bone Malignancies

Paul W. Gidley, MD[a],*, Franco DeMonte, MD[b]

KEYWORDS

- Temporal bone cancer • Temporal bone resection • Squamous cell carcinoma
- Basal cell carcinoma

KEY POINTS

- Squamous cell carcinoma accounts for 60% to 80% of the tumors that arise in the ear canal, middle ear, or mastoid cavity.
- Otorrhea, otalgia, and hearing loss are the most common symptoms of temporal bone tumors and can be confused with benign disease.
- Preoperative staging requires computed tomography, magnetic resonance imaging, or both. The University of Pittsburgh staging system is useful for treatment planning and prognostication.
- Lateral temporal bone resection is required to treat most tumors. Auriculectomy, parotidectomy, mandibulectomy, craniotomy, and neck dissection are performed based on staging and location of tumor. Temporalis muscle flap or microvascular free flap are reconstruction options.
- Adjuvant radiotherapy is recommended for temporal bone tumors staged T2 and higher. Adjuvant chemotherapy has an emerging role for T3 and T4 tumors.

EPIDEMIOLOGY

Primary tumors that affect the temporal bone are rare. Primary ear canal cancers or middle ear cancers occur at an estimated rate of 1 person per million people per year.[1–3] It is estimated that cancer is the underlying cause in only 1 in every 5000 to 20,000 patients with an otologic complaint.[4] Temporal bone carcinomas account for only about 0.2% of all head and neck cancers.[5] Sun exposure is linked with skin cancers, and radiotherapy has been linked with squamous cell cancer of middle ear and ear canal.[6] Some investigators have linked chronic otitis media and cholesteatoma to ear canal and middle ear cancer,[6–9] but this cause probably accounts for only a few tumors in most modern studies. For most patients, the cause is unknown.

Because primary ear canal and middle ear cancers are so rare, the temporal bone is more likely to be affected secondarily from advanced periauricular skin cancer or the parotid gland tumors than from primary tumors.[10]

Tumors affecting the temporal bone can occur in all age groups, but typically occur in older patients, especially in men. In a large series of temporal bone cancers, 75% of patients were men, and the average age was 65 years.[11] The tumor histologies tend to trend with age, so that younger patients are likely to have sarcomas and older patients are likely to have carcinomas.

SIGNS AND SYMPTOMS

The signs and symptoms of these tumors are vague and can be confused with benign disease. Otorrhea, otalgia, and hearing loss are the most common symptoms of temporal bone tumors.[12] However, these symptoms are frequently seen in patients with otitis externa, otitis media, or cholesteatoma. Most patients with benign disease respond to aural toilet and eardrops or oral

Funding sources: None.
Conflict of interest: None.
[a] Department of Head and Neck Surgery, The University of Texas MD Anderson Cancer Center, 1515 Holcombe Boulevard, Unit 1445, Houston, TX 77030, USA; [b] Department of Neurosurgery, The University of Texas MD Anderson Cancer Center, 1515 Holcombe Boulevard, Unit 442, Houston, TX 77030, USA
* Corresponding author.
E-mail address: pwgidley@mdanderson.org

neurosurgery.theclinics.com

medications. Suspicion should arise when patients with these symptoms do not respond to standard therapy.

Otorrhea, otalgia, and hearing loss make up a classic triad for temporal bone cancer, but this classic triad is seen in only 10% of patients who have temporal bone cancer. Other symptoms, such as trismus, facial weakness, dysphagia, and hoarseness, are seen less commonly and are usually associated with advanced-stage disease.

The duration of symptoms can vary from months to several years.[12,13] Survival has been linked to symptom duration.[13] For this reason, a high index of suspicion should be maintained when symptoms do not resolve with standard therapy for benign diseases.

The physical examination of these patients demands close scrutiny of the external ear, ear canals, tympanic membranes, parotid gland, periauricular skin, cervical lymph nodes, and cranial nerves. Microscopic examination of the ear canal is important to determine the extent of disease into the ear canal. Tumors of the external ear that do not extend medially past the bony-cartilaginous junction in the ear canal can often be dealt with by local excision. However, tumors that involve the bony ear canal require, at a minimum, lateral temporal bone resection (LTBR) to achieve a negative medial margin.

Skin cancers involving the ear canal have an exophytic or ulcerated appearance (**Fig. 1**).

Squamous cell carcinoma (SCCa) can be heralded by erythematous skin and granulation tissue. Basal cell carcinoma usually has an ulcerated appearance with rolled edges. Adenoid cystic carcinoma (ACCa) in its early stage is often subcutaneous. Occasionally, some tumors have a subcutaneous spread and a cursory examination of the canal might miss the ear canal involvement (**Fig. 2**).

When patients with these symptoms do not respond to standard therapy, then any suspicious tissue should be sent for pathologic evaluation. The differential diagnosis for disease in the ear canal should include skull base osteomyelitis (also called malignant otitis externa), pseudoepitheliamotous hyperplasia, and carcinoma.[14] The temporal bone and ear canal are a rare location for metastatic lesions, usually from breast, lung, or kidney primaries.[15,16]

Facial paralysis, when it occurs, it is an ominous finding. It is linked with a poor prognosis.[17] In a series from MD Anderson Cancer Center, approximately 40% of patients had various degrees of facial weakness or paralysis at presentation.[11]

Cervical lymphadenopathy is a particularly poor prognostic sign associated with worse survival.

LOCATION OF PRIMARY TUMOR

Primary tumors of the ear canal or temporal bone are rare. In our patient population, those 2 primary sites account for only 25% of our total patient population (**Fig. 3**).[11] Instead, the temporal bone is more likely to be invaded by cancers of the parotid

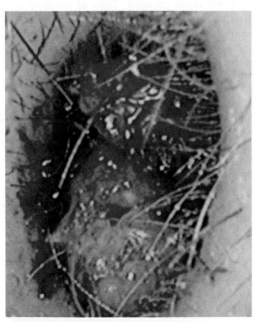

Fig. 1. Squamous cell carcinoma filling the left ear canal. (*From* the Department of Head and Neck Surgery, MD Anderson Cancer Center; with permission.)

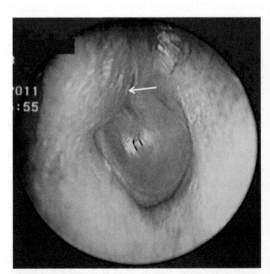

Fig. 2. Subtle left anterior-superior ear canal swelling (*arrow*) caused by infratemporal fossa chondrosarcomas. (*From* the Department of Head and Neck Surgery, MD Anderson Cancer Center; with permission.)

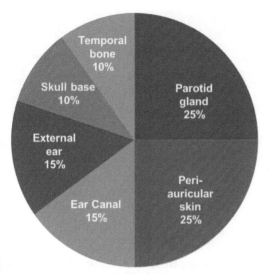

Fig. 3. Location of temporal bone primary tumors. (*From* the Department of Head and Neck Surgery, MD Anderson Cancer Center; with permission.)

gland or periauricular skin. These 2 primary sites combine for 50% of our temporal bone patient population. Advanced, neglected external ear cancers that have grown into the ear canal and skull-based cancers, primarily sarcomas, make up the remaining 25% of our patient population.

HISTOLOGY

A long list of tumor types has been described as affecting the temporal bone (**Box 1**).[11] Squamous cell and basal cell carcinoma account for more than 50% of the tumors if all primary tumor sites are considered. When primary locations outside the temporal bone are excluded, SCCa accounts for 60% to 80% of the tumors that arise in the ear canal, middle ear, or mastoid cavity.[18–20] Basal cell carcinoma and ACCa are the next 2 most common tumors found in the ear canal.

DIAGNOSTIC IMAGING

Diagnostic imaging is imperative for understanding the three-dimensional anatomy of these tumors. Computed tomography (CT) and magnetic resonance imaging (MRI) provide complimentary details.[21] A CT scan is generally obtained as an initial study. It gives an excellent view of soft tissue and bony anatomy. Because surgery is the mainstay of temporal bone cancer treatment, the bony anatomy is especially important for temporal bone surgeons. A high-riding jugular bulb and anomalous carotid artery are important to recognize and are readily identifiable on CT imaging (**Figs. 4** and **5**).

Box 1
List of malignant tumor types found affecting the temporal bone

Epithelial
SCCa
Basal cell carcinoma
ACCa
Basosquamous carcinoma
Hidradenocarcinoma
Melanoma
Sarcomatoid carcinoma
Sebaceous cell carcinoma

Sarcomas
Chondrosarcoma
Osteosarcoma
Pleomorphic sarcoma
Spindle cell sarcoma

Salivary
ACCa
Acinic cell carcinoma
Adenocarcinoma
Basal cell adenocarcinoma
Carcinoma ex-pleomorphic adenoma
Malignant mixed carcinoma
Mucoepidermoid carcinoma
Salivary ductal carcinoma

Other
Clivus chordomas
Hemangiopericytoma
Neuroendocrine carcinoma
Peripheral nerve sheath tumor

Given that MRI lacks bony detail, its use is reserved as an adjunct especially in cases in which dural involvement or perineural invasion is suspected (**Figs. 6** and **7**).

Arriaga and colleagues[22] considered 12 important sites of involvement to identify and study on CT and MRI. These sites include the 4 quadrants of the ear canal, the infratemporal fossa, middle ear, otic capsule, mastoid, jugular foramen, carotid canal, tegmen, middle fossa, and posterior fossa.

Leonetti and colleagues[23] looked at different paths of invasion of temporal bone tumors. They identified that tumors grow superiorly through the tegmen, anteriorly through the glenoid fossa and

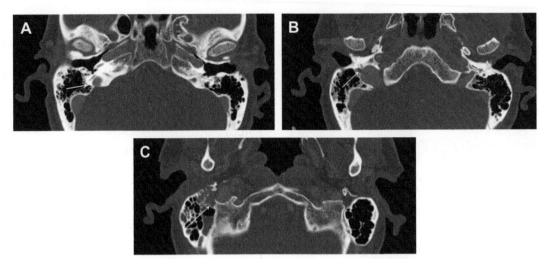

Fig. 4. CT of right parotid tumor with perineural invasion of facial nerve destroying stylomastoid foramen. (*A*) High-riding jugular bulb present at level of posterior semicircular canal (*arrow*). (*B*) Facial canal contiguous with jugular bulb (*arrow*). (*C*) Stylomastoid foramen destroyed by tumor. (*From* the Department of Head and Neck Surgery, MD Anderson Cancer Center; with permission.)

infratemporal space, inferiorly through the hypotympanum and jugular foramen, posteriorly into the mastoid, and medially through the carotid canal and inner ear. They noted that anterior and inferior spread is accurately assessed by CT scan and MRI; however, they found that there was underestimation of disease when it involved mastoid and middle ear mucosa, the tegmen tympani, the middle fossa dural, or the carotid canal. Local recurrences were found in these 4 areas on retrospective review.[23]

No staging system has been approved for temporal bone cancers by the American Joint Committee on Cancer. Several staging systems have been proposed.[3,24–27] The first iteration of the University of Pittsburgh staging system was proposed by Arriaga and colleagues[25] in 1990 and was modified more recently by Moody and colleagues[5] (**Table 1**). This staging system provides a comprehensive means of assessing these tumors, and the Pittsburgh T stage has been shown to predict overall survival.[12]

Early-stage T1 tumors are limited to the ear canal without any bony erosion or soft tissue involvement. T2 tumors have limited ear canal bony erosion or limited soft tissue involvement.

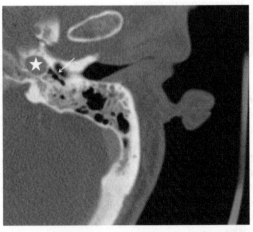

Fig. 5. CT of left temporal bone showing inferior bony annulus (*arrow*) at level of carotid canal (*star*). Patient has large parotid tumor necessitating LTBR. (*From* the Department of Head and Neck Surgery, MD Anderson Cancer Center; with permission.)

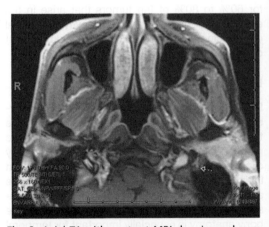

Fig. 6. Axial T1 with contrast MRI showing enhancement of intratemporal facial nerve (*arrow*) caused by perineural invasion from parotid tumor. (*From* the Department of Head and Neck Surgery, MD Anderson Cancer Center; with permission.)

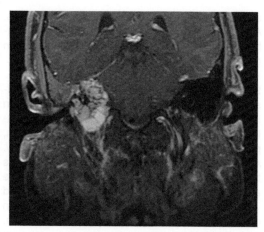

Fig. 7. Coronal T1 enhanced MRI of large right endo-lymphatic sac tumor showing tumor largely contained by the dura. (*From* the Department of Head and Neck Surgery, MD Anderson Cancer Center; with permission.)

T3 tumors are larger tumors that erode the bony ear canal or have limited soft tissue involvement or begin to involve the middle ear or mastoid. T4 are large tumors that involve the inner ear, the carotid canal, the jugular foramen, and the dura or have evidence of facial paresis. The presence of facial paralysis is an important change in the current system of staging when compared with the original iteration.[28]

Given that cervical lymphadenopathy carries a poor prognosis, overall staging for temporal bone tumors is different from staging for other head and neck tumor sites. T1N0 tumors are stage 1, T2N0 tumors are stage 2, and T3N0 tumors are stage 3. However, stage 4 tumors include T4N0 and any T with N+ status.[25]

TREATMENT: SURGERY

Although single modality radiotherapy has been reported as a treatment of temporal bone tumors,[29–31] surgical resection has been considered the standard of care. Surgical management of these tumors is predicated on and tailored to the extent of disease. The goal of surgery is to extirpate disease, achieving a negative margin and minimizing morbidity or mortality.

Local Canal Excision

Small, early staged tumors that are confined to the cartilaginous outer ear canal can be managed with a wide local excision.[19] This situation occasionally arises in the case of a tragal-based or conchal-based tumor that extends into the membranous ear canal. This procedure is usually performed under general anesthesia using the operative microscope. An endaural incision helps with

Table 1
Modified Pittsburgh staging system[5] for SCCa of the temporal bone

T Classification	Description
T1	Limited to the EAC without bony erosion or evidence of soft tissue involvement
T2	Limited to the EAC with bone erosion (not full thickness) or limited soft tissue involvement (<0.5 cm)
T3	Erosion through the osseous EAC (full thickness), with limited soft tissue involvement (<0.5 cm) or tumor involvement in the middle ear or mastoid
T4	Erosion of the cochlea, petrous apex, medial wall of the middle ear, carotid canal, jugular foramen, or dura, with extensive soft tissue involvement (>0.5 cm, such as involvement of the TMJ or styloid process), or evidence of facial paresis
N classification	
N0	No regional nodes involved
N1	Single metastatic regional node <3 cm
N2	
N2a	Single ipsilateral metastatic node 3–6 cm
N2b	Multiple ipsilateral metastatic lymph nodes
N2c	Contralateral metastatic lymph node
N3	Metastatic lymph node >6 cm
Overall Stage	
I	T1N0
II	T2N0
III	T3N0
IV	T4N0 and T1-4N+

Abbreviations: EAC, external auditory canal; N+, any positive lymph node; TMJ, temporomandibular joint.

visualizing tumor extent. Skin and underlying cartilage are excised using frozen-section pathology for margin evaluation. Reconstruction is performed with a split-thickness skin graft.

The skin of the bony ear canal is thin, and achieving a negative deep margin is difficult once the tumor reaches the bony ear canal. If the medial (or bony canal) extent of the tumor cannot be cleared, then the procedure should be converted to an LTBR. Anecdotally, surgeons have tried to remove the skin from the bony ear canal, the so-called sleeve resection, reconstructed the defect with a split-thickness skin graft and used radiotherapy as a salvage therapy. This situation usually develops into a narrow ear canal with exposed bone and chronic drainage and can lead to osteoradionecrosis of the temporal bone. LTBR provides better tumor control and overall survival for these patients.

LTBR

The real workhorse of otologic oncologic surgery is the LTBR. This procedure removes the bony canal en bloc lateral to the facial nerve (**Fig. 8**). The specimen includes the tympanic membrane, malleus, and incus. The stapes, facial nerve, and inner ear structures are preserved. The amount of cartilaginous ear canal and pinna resected depends on the tumor extent in these structures. LTBR can be combined with parotidectomy, neck dissection, mandibulectomy, and craniotomy. Reconstruction technique depends on the defect and is influenced by previous irradiation.

General considerations LTBR with parotidectomy, neck dissection, and possible microvascular free-flap reconstruction usually requires 8 to 12 hours of general anesthesia. The patient's general health must allow such a surgical procedure. Intraoperative facial nerve monitoring is always used, and this fact must be communicated to the

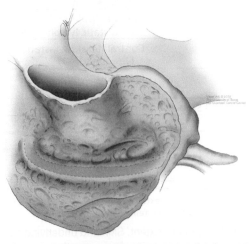

Fig. 8. Line facial nerve dissection as part of right LTBR. (*From* the Department of Head and Neck Surgery, MD Anderson Cancer Center; with permission.)

anesthetist to avoid use of long-term paralytics. Antithromboembolism techniques, thromboembolic deterrent hoses, and sequential compression devices are also used.

Skin incision The surgeon has a choice of incisions for temporal bone resection. This decision is based on location of tumor, the need for auriculectomy, parotidectomy or neck dissection, previous incisions, and the need for craniotomy. A large postauricular C-shaped incision is perhaps the most versatile incision and is used when the auricle is normal. The auricle can be elevated with a wide anteriorly based skin flap. This incision gives access for parotidectomy, neck dissection, and craniotomy.

When auriculectomy is required, an incision that circumscribes the tumor and auricle is used. Surrounding skin can be undermined, giving enough exposure for LTBR, parotidectomy, and neck dissection. Limited middle fossa craniectomy can be performed through this approach. This situation produces the largest soft tissue defect and generally requires a microvascular free flap for closure.

When the tumor is confined to the ear canal, a modified parotidectomy incision can be combined with an elliptical incision around the external meatus. This incision is especially advantageous in the circumstance of recurrent disease after previous parotidectomy. The incision can be extended anterior to the helix and superiorly into the temporal scalp. The remaining pinna is elevated with a broad posteriorly based skin flap. This incision is probably best for T1 and T2 ear canal cancers and parotid-based tumors that involve the ear canal. Parotidectomy and neck dissection are performed, and reconstruction can be with either a temporalis muscle flap or a microvascular free flap. The posteriorly based skin flap containing the pinna has some disadvantages: (1) the pinna is folded or retracted, which could compromise its blood supply, and (2) the surgeon has to work over the flap containing the pinna.

Bony dissection The goal of LTBR is en bloc resection of tumors involving the external auditory canal. The strategy to achieve this goal is bony dissection to free the external canal. After skin incisions, a complete mastoidectomy is performed. The tegmen is thinned and used as a guide to judge the level of the middle fossa dura. The antrum is opened, the attic is widened, and the incus and malleus head are identified. The horizontal semicircular canal is preserved throughout this dissection.

Bone at the root of the zygoma is removed, and the temporomandibular joint is identified at its lateral bony margin. Drilling continues through zygomatic air cells, working lateral to the ossicular chain and between the bony ear canal and the tegmen. Care is taken to avoid a dural tear. Equally, care is taken to avoid violating the external ear canal bone and spilling tumor into the operative field. This dissection is complete when the entire temporomandibular joint capsule is exposed from medial to lateral.

The facial recess is opened, and the middle ear is checked for disease. (If disease is found in the middle ear, the surgical procedure needs to expand beyond an LTBR.) The facial nerve is identified at its tympanic segment and followed through its mastoid course to the stylomastoid foramen. The digastric ridge is drilled away to identify the underlying digastric muscle. A cut is made in the anterior wall of the mastoid tip, lateral to the facial nerve and inferior to the tympanic ring. This maneuver liberates the mastoid tip, and its soft tissue attachments are cut with electrocautery. Removal of the mastoid tip unifies the mastoid with the neck, and it allows the facial nerve to be traced from the mastoid into the parotid gland.

The facial recess is then extended, and the chorda tympani nerve is divided. The annulus is identified, and drilling continues between the annulus and the facial nerve until the hypotympanum is reached. The inferior tympanic bone is removed, and the soft tissue anterior to the tympanic ring is identified. In making the inferior final cut, care must be exercised to avoid having the shaft of the drill rest on the facial nerve. Only prudent surgical technique can avoid injury to the facial nerve here, because the facial nerve monitor does not alarm because injury to the facial nerve from the drill shaft is thermal.

The final bony cuts are made to free the anterior-inferior extent of the tympanic ring. Occasionally, the carotid artery is in contact with the annulus here. Vigilance is required to avoid injury to a laterally placed carotid artery.

The incus is disarticulated. Thumb pressure on the canal causes it to fracture anteriorly. A Freer elevator can be used to ensure that the canal is entirely mobilized, but care must be taken to avoid using the facial canal or middle fossa dura as a fulcrum.

Facial nerve management The mastoid segment of the facial nerve can be decompressed, and the nerve traced into the parotid gland. The facial nerve can be assessed for perineural disease. Perineural disease can produce a nerve that is thicker and redder than usual. If the patient has normal facial function preoperatively, then efforts should be made to preserve this function. If the patient has preexisting facial paralysis and facial nerve sacrifice is planned, then the nerve can be divided and the proximal end sent for frozen-section evaluation. A tumor-free margin should be sought; however, a labyrinthectomy is not performed for the reason of trying to achieve a negative facial nerve margin. Our philosophy has been to treat this remaining microscopic disease with postoperative radiotherapy. Successful facial nerve grafting and reasonable survival can be achieved even when microscopic disease remains in the proximal segment of the facial nerve.[32]

If nerve sacrifice is required and if usable proximal and distal segments are available, then an attempt should be made at facial nerve grafting.[33,34] The great auricular nerve is a reasonable choice for short defects; however, the facial nerve defects that result from LTBR and parotidectomy are usually too long to be grafted with the greater auricular nerve. Sural nerve and the cutaneous branch of the anterior femoral nerve, which is in the field of the anterior lateral thigh flap, are better options.[33]

Some tumors can be adequately treated with LTBR alone; however, most cases require concomitant parotidectomy and upper neck dissection (level II and III). These procedures commence after LTBR. Large auricular cancers and large parotid tumors can be resected en bloc along with the ear canal. This surgery creates a composite resection that includes the external ear, ear canal, parotid, and neck dissection and occasionally the upper mandible as 1 single specimen (**Fig. 9**).

Reconstruction Historically, surgeons reconstructed the lateral temporal bone defect by covering the cavity with a split-thickness skin graft.[35] This technique offered patients an option for hearing reconstruction. However, these cavities can develop serious, bothersome drainage and infection, especially after radiotherapy. Furthermore, these patients tended to have poor hearing outcomes, given the possible chronic infection and sensorineural hearing loss from radiotherapy.

More modern techniques of reconstruction emphasize closing off the cavity from the outside world. The type of reconstruction depends on several factors: size of defect, history of preoperative radiotherapy, vascular and dural coverage, and cosmesis. Small, uncomplicated defects can be reconstructed with temporalis muscle flap.[36] A split-thickness skin graft can be used to cover the flap and to close a small cutaneous defect. However, microvascular free-flap reconstruction is required in most circumstances, especially in

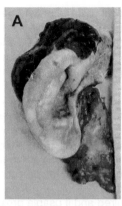
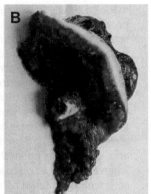
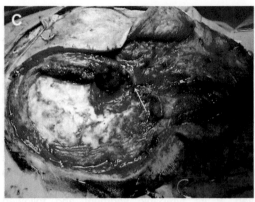

Fig. 9. Surgical specimen and defect after composite temporal bone resection. (*A*) Lateral surface showing large periauricular tumor. (*B*) Medial surface of specimen showing intact ear canal and eardrum. (*C*) Surgical defect after total auriculectomy, LTBR, neck dissection, and parotidectomy. Note the course of the facial nerve (*arrow*). This defect was closed with an anterolateral thigh flap. (*From* the Department of Head and Neck Surgery, MD Anderson Cancer Center; with permission.)

patients with large skin defects or previous radiotherapy or when the dura or vascular structures need coverage.[34,37,38]

When facial nerve sacrifice has occurred, techniques for facial rehabilitation and eye protection should be considered at the time of the primary surgery. Gold weights, tarsorrhaphy, canthoplasty, brow lifts, and static slings each have a role to play. Oculoplastic surgeons are invaluable members of the team to help manage eye complications related to facial paralysis.

Osseointegrated implants offer patients an option for hearing restoration and for prosthesis fixation. Implants can be placed either at the time of primary surgery or at a time after completion of therapy. Loading can begin in 3 months in patients not treated with radiotherapy. However, 6 months are allowed to pass before using an implant in an irradiated field.

Subtotal temporal bone resection

Tumors that extend into the middle ear need surgery beyond the LTBR.[26] Subtotal temporal bone resection (STBR) extends the dissection into the labyrinth, the cochlea, or both. Often, LTBR is required as an initial first step to permit access to deeper structures.

Skin incisions These tumors tend to have their epicenter in the middle ear or mastoid and thus have limited ear canal involvement. A large C-shaped postauricular incision works well. Frozen section is used to confirm a negative ear canal margin, and the ear canal is oversewn.

Bony dissection LTBR is performed to remove the disease contained within the ear canal. This procedure gives an unimpeded view of the middle ear,

inner ear, and carotid-jugular triangle. Dissection is directed by disease extension. Labyrinthectomy, jugular foramen dissection, and cochlectomy are performed as needed depending on disease extent. The eustachian tube mucosa can be involved, and the carotid artery often must be dissected and decompressed. Tumor dissection is performed in a piecemeal fashion. Tissue sampling for frozen section is used liberally to determine the full extent of disease.

The dura of either the posterior or middle fossa is often involved in these tumors. Dural resection is again directed by extent of disease, and frozen section is used to control the margin.

Facial nerve management These patients generally present with facial nerve dysfunction, and these tumors generally involve the facial nerve in its mastoid or tympanic segments. Facial nerve sacrifice is required in this circumstance. Because labyrinthectomy is being performed, the facial nerve can be traced proximally and a tumor-free margin can be obtained. Occasionally, a low-grade tumor, such as an endolymphatic sac tumor or middle ear neuroendocrine tumor, can be adequately dissected away from the nerve and facial function preserved.

Reconstruction techniques These procedures generally do not produce large cutaneous defects, but reconstruction is complicated by the presence of a dural defect and the potential for cerebrospinal fluid (CSF) leak. A water-tight dural repair should be attempted using allograft duraplasty, but this can be impossible for some defects. Overlay temporalis fascia and abdominal fat graft, as is used in acoustic neuroma surgery, is another option for a small dural defect. Microvascular free flaps can be used, especially in the setting of previous radiotherapy.

Total temporal bone resection

Although en bloc total temporal bone resection has been reported,[39–42] our team does not use this technique. Carotid resection is common to en bloc total temporal bone resection (TTBR), and this carries with it a high morbidity. Our philosophy has been to avoid carotid artery resection for malignant disease, because it produces significant morbidity and does not carry an improvement in overall disease-free survival.

TTBR extends the dissection as described earlier for STBR and includes removal of the internal auditory canal and petrous apex. Disease removal is piecemeal and directed by frozen-section pathology. Reconstruction considerations are similar to those described for STBR.

The role of parotidectomy and neck dissection

The parotid gland can be involved by either direct extension through the fissures of Santorini or by metastatic spread to intraparotid lymph nodes.[19,43] Morris and colleagues[19] described a series of 72 patients with temporal bone cancer, 36% of whom had direct tumor invasion into the parotid and 25% of whom had metastatic intraparotid lymph nodes. Gidley and colleagues[11] found that about 11% of their series of 157 patients with temporal bone cancer had salivary gland invasion. For these reasons, superficial parotidectomy, at a minimum, should be performed with LTBR.

Primary tumors of the ear canal, middle ear, and mastoid rarely (around 10%) present with cervical lymphadenopathy.[19,44–46] Level II and III are most commonly involved.[11] Although overall nodal involvement is low, neck dissection and parotidectomy permit accurate tumor staging.[12,47] Neck dissection also facilitates vessel exposure when microvascular free-flap reconstruction is needed.

Because the ear canal is more commonly involved by parotid primaries or periauricular skin cancers, parotidectomy and neck dissection are required to address the primary tumor.[48]

Complications of surgery

Temporal bone resection can be associated with high complication rates. All patients are counseled about the risks of surgery: hearing loss, tinnitus, dizziness, facial weakness or paralysis, loss of taste on the tongue, loss of the outer ear, CSF leak, and meningitis. Major complications, defined as requiring additional surgery or additional intensive medical therapy, have remained less than 10%. CSF leak and meningitis occur at rates consistent with transtemporal skull base surgery.

Pulmonary embolism, myocardial infarction, and death have been reported after temporal bone resection.[11,49] For these reasons, patients must be in good general health to be able to tolerate such surgery.

A maximal conductive hearing loss is the expected side effect of LTBR. This hearing loss can be overcome with an osseointegrated bone conducting hearing aid. Single-sided deafness occurs from STBR and TTBR. Osseointegrated bone conducting hearing aids and a contralateral routing of sound hearing aid are options for hearing rehabilitation for these patients.

Facial paralysis is a disappointing, but often unavoidable, outcome of temporal bone surgery. Rates of facial nerve sacrifice might be nearly 50%.[11] Plastic reconstructive surgeons and oculoplastic surgeons are invaluable in helping to manage facial paralysis, to restore cosmesis, and to protect vision.

Contraindications to surgery

Surgery is not indicated for patients with unresectable disease, distant metastasis, or poor general health status. Tumors that encase the carotid or vertebral artery, that erode into the cervical spine, or that have significant brain invasion are not considered for surgical treatment. Although the use of carotid artery bypass has been reported for skull base cancers,[50] the long-term results for this technique are disappointing, yielding only a 20% 2-year survival and the attendant risks of postoperative stroke or death.[51] Our team has avoided such surgery and relied on palliative chemotherapy and radiotherapy for these patients.

Isolated and limited temporal lobe involvement can be resected.[41,52] Moffat and colleagues[53,54] have reported reasonable results after resection of temporal bone tumors with brain invasion. However, in our patient population, we have rarely found isolated brain invasion from temporal bone tumors that did not have concomitant carotid artery involvement or metastatic disease.[11]

TREATMENT: RADIOTHERAPY

Radiotherapy plays a significant role as adjuvant therapy for temporal bone cancers or as a treatment of patients who are not candidates for surgery. Primary radiotherapy was used to treat temporal bone cancers up to the 1970s[20,55,56]; however, this technique had a low overall cure rate. Only a few articles have reviewed the role of radiotherapy as single modality therapy. Kang and colleagues[57] concluded that radiotherapy alone was not inferior to combined surgery and radiotherapy for disease-specific survival (DSS), but they found that local control was worse when radiotherapy alone was used.

Advances in skull base techniques vaulted surgery into its current role as primary therapy, using radiotherapy as a postoperative adjuvant.[19,58] The combination of these 2 modalities has improved overall survival for patients who have temporal bone cancer.[9,38]

Currently, radiotherapy is recommended for T2 and higher staged tumors.[12,54,59,60] Other indications for postoperative radiotherapy include recurrent tumors, positive margins, perineural spread, positive lymph nodes, or extracapsular spread.[38]

Intensity modulated radiotherapy (IMRT) allows the radiation oncologist the ability to adequately treat the tumor site and minimize dose to surrounding structures, especially the temporal lobe and brainstem. Dosages vary widely in the literature. Pfreundner and colleagues[61] recommended 54 to 60 Gy in patients with negative margins and a minimum of 66 Gy with positive margins. Prabhu and colleagues[62] gave doses between 60 and 66 Gy for patients with negative margins and doses between 68 and 72 Gy for patients with positive or close margins.

TREATMENT: CHEMOTHERAPY

Advancements in chemotherapeutic agents have ushered in a new era for head and neck tumors.[63–68] Data from these studies have been extrapolated from mucosal epithelial tumors of the head and neck to other sites. Only a few isolated studies have examined the role of chemotherapy for temporal bone cancers.[69–71]

Nakagawa and colleagues[69] described a series of 25 patients with primary SCCa of the ear canal and middle ear. Six patients (T2: 1 patient; T3: 3 patients; T4: 2 patients) received preoperative chemotherapy followed by surgery and radiotherapy. Five of these 6 patients achieved mean survival of 60 months. Chemotherapy and radiotherapy alone were used in 7 patients with T4 disease; 3 of these 7 patients had no evidence of disease at mean of 31.6 months.

In a pilot study, Shiga and colleagues[70] described a series of 14 patients with SCCa of the temporal bone, of whom 9 had stage IV disease and were treated with concomitant chemoradiotherapy. Their chemotherapy regimen included docetaxel, cisplatin, and 5-fluorouracil (TPF). Eight of 9 patients achieved complete response. These investigators concluded that the use of concomitant chemotherapy with TPF was safe and effective as a treatment of patients with cancer of the temporal bone.[70]

Intra-arterial chemotherapy has been proposed and tested in a few patients. Sugimoto and colleagues[71] published a small series of 5 patients with T3 and T4 SCCa of the temporal bone who were treated with radiotherapy and intra-arterial chemotherapy consisting of cisplatin and thiosulfate. Three patients obtained a complete response and had mean survival of 28 months.

OUTCOMES: RECURRENCE AND SURVIVAL

Historically, temporal bone tumors were associated with dismal results and a poor prognosis.[72,73] However, advancements in multiplanar imaging, skull base surgical techniques, IMRT, and chemotherapy have combined to improve overall survival. A cogent staging system, as proposed initially by Arriaga and colleagues[25] and later modified by Moody and colleagues,[5] has allowed comparison of results across time and institutions. This later iteration of the Pittsburgh staging has shown that survival is progressively worse with increasing T stage,[17] and this finding is supported by other studies.[12,45,74] The Pittsburgh tumor staging is an important, independent factor for prognosis, and a reliable predictor for outcomes for SCCa.[12]

Small tumors that are limited to the ear canal with minimal soft tissue involvement or bone erosion (ie, T1 and T2 tumors) can be completely excised with LTBR. Whereas T1 tumors can be treated with surgery alone, T2 tumors have improved outcomes when postoperative radiotherapy is added.[12,60] Those patients with early-stage disease have 80% to 100% 5-year survival rates.[7,75,76]

Larger tumors (T3 and T4) involve significantly more anatomic structures and present a significantly more difficult tumor to treat. These tumors can be conceptualized in 2 varieties: external ear canal tumors that erode past the eardrum into the middle ear, or tumors that arise primarily within the middle ear, inner ear, or mastoid. When tumors involve the middle ear, the LTBR is no longer an adequate or sufficient surgical treatment.[77] Multidisciplinary team management is required for these larger, advanced-stage tumors. These patients might require a combination of surgery, radiotherapy, and chemotherapy for treatment of their tumors. Treatment goals remain consistent despite the large size of the tumor: adequate disease resection to achieve negative margin and minimizing damage to surrounding normal structures. Despite adequate treatment, overall 5-year survival rates do not exceed 50% for this group of late-stage tumors (**Table 2**).

Facial nerve involvement, positive lymph nodes, extratemporal disease extension, and positive

Table 2
Comparison of recently published survival results for SCCa of the ear canal and temporal bone. Only studies with 20 or more patients are included

Authors, Year	Total Patients (n)	T Stage[a] (n)	Mean Fu (mo)	Overall 5-y Survival (%)	DSS (%)	Disease-Free Survival (%)
Yin et al,[45] 2006	95	NS	NS	66.8 (cohort) Stage I = 100 Stage II = 100 Stage III = 67.2 Stage IV = 29.5	NS	NS
Nakagawa et al,[69] 2006	25	T1 = 1 T2 = 3 T3 = 5 T4 = 16	39	T1 and T2 = 80 (estimated) T3 and T4 = 40 (estimated)	NS	NS
Kunst et al,[79] 2008	28	pT1 = 12 pT2 = 2 pT3 = 4 pT4 = 10	34	64 (cohort) T1 = 83 T4 = 25	NS	NS
Madsen et al,[74] 2008	47	T1 = 13 T2 = 7 T3 = 7 T4 = 19	48	31	42%	NS
Kang et al,[57] 2009	35	T1 = 10* T2 = 11 T3 = 14	34	NS	80 (3-y)	63 (3-y)
Prabhu et al,[62] 2009	30	T1 = 7* T2 = 5 T3 = 18	24	54	T1 and T2 = 70 T3 = 41	T1 and T2 = 73 T3 = 55
Gidley et al,[12] 2010	71	T1 = 20 T2 = 15 T3 = 5 T4 = 31	NS	38	NS	60
Chi et al,[7] 2011	72	T1 = 15 T2 = 3 T3 = 19 T4 = 35	NS	T1 = 100 T2 = 66.7 T3 = 21.1 T4 = 14.3	NS	NS

[a] Pittsburgh 2000 staging system[5] is used except where noted by an asterisk for Stell and McCormack staging system.[24]

surgical margins are all factors linked with poor overall survival.[6,7,11,19,45,74] Higgins and Moody[17] performed a systematic review of SCCa of the temporal bone to examine the effect of facial paralysis on survival outcomes. Their pooled data showed 5-year overall survival of 19.1% in patients with facial paralysis versus 59.4% in patients without facial paralysis, regardless of tumor stage.

Although lymph node metastases are uncommon, their presence is a significant risk factor for poor survival.[11] For patients with SCCa, Morris and colleagues[19] reported that 5-year DSS was 81% in node-negative patients and 19% in node-positive patients (P<.0001). A stark contrast in survival was also reported by Gidley and colleagues.[11]

Margin status is a strong predictor for recurrence, and rates of positive margins vary between 20% and 33%.[7,11,12,19,45,74] Morris and colleagues[19] describe 5-year DSS of 81.7% for patients with negative margins versus 50.0% for patients with positive margins (P = .03, long rank).

Other factors that are linked to high recurrence rates and poor survival include middle ear invasion,[74] need for mandibulectomy,[11,19] performance of craniotomy, facial nerve sacrifice, and parapharyngeal space or infratemporal fossa dissection.[78] Middle ear invasion is an important factor, because tumors that are confined to the ear canal can be resected en bloc with LTBR. Survival rates decrease to about 20% when the middle ear is involved with tumor, compared with 60% or higher when the middle ear is not involved.[20,74]

Intracranial disease extension can be successfully treated.[49,54] Dural involvement was seen in about 5% of patients from a series of 157 patients with temporal bone cancer reported by Gidley and colleagues.[11] Dean and colleagues[38] found intracranial disease in 16 of 65 patients, and they found that it did not have an effect on disease-free survival. The local control rates were similar with or without intracranial extension (76.9% vs 71.7%, respectively).[38]

Recurrences tend to occur within the first 2 years after completion of therapy.[11,19] A large study of 157 patients with temporal bone tumors showed a mean time to recurrence of 13 months.[11] In this study, recurrences were 12.7% local, 6.4% regional, and 13.4% distant. The most common sites for distant spread are lung, brain, and dermal metastases.[11] Morris and colleagues[19] showed recurrence rates of 20.5% for local disease, 5.5% for regional disease, and 22.9% for distant disease. Recurrence rates tended to be higher with salivary gland origin tumors.

Because temporal bone tumors are rare, many investigators have lumped several different tumor histologies into analysis.[11,19] This lumping can make analysis difficult because tumor biology and behavior vary widely among these histologies. A clear distinction in tumor behavior exists between SCCa and ACCa. Although SCCa is the most common tumor type, it has a lower overall 5-year survival rate than is reported for ACCa of the ear canal.[12,13] Although mean time to recurrence with SCCa is around 2 years, the mean time to recurrence for ACCa is reported to be nearly 8 years.[12,13]

SUMMARY

Primary temporal bone tumors are rare, and the temporal bone is more likely to be involved secondarily by tumors from the parotid gland or periauricular skin. Ear canal cancers are rare and do not have specific symptoms distinguishing them from benign ear canal conditions. Suspicious lesions of the ear canal should be biopsied for proper diagnosis. The most common tumor type is squamous cell cancer; however, a long list of tumor types have been described involving the temporal bone.

Surgical resection to achieve negative margins is the mainstay of treatment. Small tumors (T1 and T2) can often be treated with LTBR. Parotidectomy and neck dissection are added for disease extension and proper staging. Higher staged tumors, T3 and T4, generally require STBR or TTBR along with possible craniotomy, mandibulectomy, resection of the zygoma, and dissection of the infratemporal fossa.

Small defects can be adequately reconstructed with a temporalis muscle flap. Microvascular free flaps are used for large defects and for patients with a history of previous radiotherapy. Adjuvant postoperative radiotherapy has shown improved survival for patients with tumors staged T2 or higher. Chemotherapy has an emerging role for advanced-stage disease. Evaluation and management of patients with temporal bone tumors by a multidisciplinary team are critical to optimize outcomes in this group of patients.

REFERENCES

1. Clark LJ, Narula AA, Morgan DA, et al. Squamous carcinoma of the temporal bone: a revised staging. J Laryngol Otol 1991;105(5):346–8.
2. Morton RP, Stell PM, Derrick PP. Epidemiology of cancer of the middle ear cleft. Cancer 1984;53(7): 1612–7.
3. Arena S, Keen M. Carcinoma of the middle ear and temporal bone. Am J Otol 1988;9(5):351–6.
4. Conley JJ. Cancer of the middle ear and temporal bone. N Y State J Med 1974;74(9):1575–9.
5. Moody SA, Hirsch BE, Myers EN. Squamous cell carcinoma of the external auditory canal: an evaluation of a staging system. Am J Otol 2000;21(4):582–8.
6. Lobo D, Llorente JL, Suarez C. Squamous cell carcinoma of the external auditory canal. Skull Base 2008;18(3):167–72.
7. Chi FL, Gu FM, Dai CF, et al. Survival outcomes in surgical treatment of 72 cases of squamous cell carcinoma of the temporal bone. Otol Neurotol 2011;32(4):665–9.
8. Rothschild S, Ciernik IF, Hartmann M, et al. Cholesteatoma triggering squamous cell carcinoma: case report and literature review of a rare tumor. Am J Otolaryngol 2009;30(4):256–60.
9. Hahn SS, Kim JA, Goodchild N, et al. Carcinoma of the middle ear and external auditory canal. Int J Radiat Oncol Biol Phys 1983;9(7):1003–7.
10. Gidley PW. Managing malignancies of the external auditory canal. Expert Rev Anticancer Ther 2009; 9(9):1277–82.
11. Gidley PW, Thompson CR, Roberts DB, et al. The oncology of otology. Laryngoscope 2012;122(2): 393–400.
12. Gidley PW, Roberts DB, Sturgis EM. Squamous cell carcinoma of the temporal bone. Laryngoscope 2010;120(6):1144–51.
13. Dong F, Gidley PW, Ho T, et al. Adenoid cystic carcinoma of the external auditory canal. Laryngoscope 2008;118(9):1591–6.
14. Gacek MR, Gacek RR, Gantz B, et al. Pseudoepitheliomatous hyperplasia versus squamous cell

carcinoma of the external auditory canal. Laryngoscope 1998;108(4 Pt 1):620–3.

15. Nelson EG, Hinojosa R. Histopathology of metastatic temporal bone tumors. Arch Otolaryngol Head Neck Surg 1991;117(2):189–93.

16. Cureoglu S, Tulunay O, Ferlito A, et al. Otologic manifestations of metastatic tumors to the temporal bone. Acta Otolaryngol 2004;124(10):1117–23.

17. Higgins TS, Antonio SA. The role of facial palsy in staging squamous cell carcinoma of the temporal bone and external auditory canal: a comparative survival analysis. Otol Neurotol 2010;31(9):1473–9.

18. Yeung P, Bridger A, Smee R, et al. Malignancies of the external auditory canal and temporal bone: a review. ANZ J Surg 2002;72(2):114–20.

19. Morris LG, Mehra S, Shah JP, et al. Predictors of survival and recurrence after temporal bone resection for cancer. Head Neck 2011;34(9):1231–9.

20. Gurgel RK, Karnell LH, Hansen MR. Middle ear cancer: a population-based study. Laryngoscope 2009;119(10):1913–7.

21. Horowitz SW, Leonetti JP, Azar-Kia B, et al. CT and MR of temporal bone malignancies primary and secondary to parotid carcinoma. AJNR Am J Neuroradiol 1994;15(4):755–62.

22. Arriaga M, Curtin HD, Takahashi H, et al. The role of preoperative CT scans in staging external auditory meatus carcinoma: radiologic-pathologic correlation study. Otolaryngol Head Neck Surg 1991;105(1):6–11.

23. Leonetti JP, Smith PG, Kletzker GR, et al. Invasion patterns of advanced temporal bone malignancies. Am J Otol 1996;17(3):438–42.

24. Stell PM, McCormick MS. Carcinoma of the external auditory meatus and middle ear. Prognostic factors and a suggested staging system. J Laryngol Otol 1985;99(9):847–50.

25. Arriaga M, Curtin H, Takahashi H, et al. Staging proposal for external auditory meatus carcinoma based on preoperative clinical examination and computed tomography findings. Ann Otol Rhinol Laryngol 1990;99(9 Pt 1):714–21.

26. Kinney SE. Squamous cell carcinoma of the external auditory canal. Am J Otol 1989;10(2):111–6.

27. Spector JG. Management of temporal bone carcinomas: a therapeutic analysis of two groups of patients and long-term followup. Otolaryngol Head Neck Surg 1991;104(1):58–66.

28. Hirsch BE. Staging system revision. Arch Otolaryngol Head Neck Surg 2002;128(1):93–4.

29. Birzgalis AR, Keith AO, Farrington WT. Radiotherapy in the treatment of middle ear and mastoid carcinoma. Clin Otolaryngol Allied Sci 1992;17(2):113–6.

30. Hashi N, Shirato H, Omatsu T, et al. The role of radiotherapy in treating squamous cell carcinoma of the external auditory canal, especially in early stages of disease. Radiother Oncol 2000;56(2):221–5.

31. Wang CC. Radiation therapy in the management of carcinoma of the external auditory canal, middle ear, or mastoid. Radiology 1975;116(3):713–5.

32. Wax MK, Kaylie DM. Does a positive neural margin affect outcome in facial nerve grafting? Head Neck 2007;29(6):546–9.

33. Gidley PW, Herrera SJ, Hanasono MM, et al. The impact of radiotherapy on facial nerve repair. Laryngoscope 2010;120(10):1985–9.

34. Hanasono MM, Silva A, Skoracki RJ, et al. Skull base reconstruction: an updated approach. Plast Reconstr Surg 2011;128(3):675–86.

35. Renton JP, Wetmore SJ. Split-thickness skin grafting in postmastoidectomy revision and in lateral temporal bone resection. Otolaryngol Head Neck Surg 2006;135(3):387–91.

36. Hanasono MM, Utley DS, Goode RL. The temporalis muscle flap for reconstruction after head and neck oncologic surgery. Laryngoscope 2001;111(10):1719–25.

37. Rosenthal EL, King T, McGrew BM, et al. Evolution of a paradigm for free tissue transfer reconstruction of lateral temporal bone defects. Head Neck 2008;30(5):589–94.

38. Dean NR, White HN, Carter DS, et al. Outcomes following temporal bone resection. Laryngoscope 2010;120(8):1516–22.

39. Sataloff RT, Myers DL, Lowry LD, et al. Total temporal bone resection for squamous cell carcinoma. Otolaryngol Head Neck Surg 1987;96(1):4–14.

40. Graham MD, Sataloff RT, Kemink JL, et al. Total en bloc resection of the temporal bone and carotid artery for malignant tumors of the ear and temporal bone. Laryngoscope 1984;94(4):528–33.

41. Okada T, Saito K, Takahashi M, et al. En bloc petrosectomy for malignant tumors involving the external auditory canal and middle ear: surgical methods and long-term outcome. J Neurosurg 2008;108(1):97–104.

42. Jimbo H, Kamata S, Miura K, et al. En bloc temporal bone resection using a diamond threadwire saw for malignant tumors. J Neurosurg 2011;114(5):1386–9.

43. Choi JY, Choi EC, Lee HK, et al. Mode of parotid involvement in external auditory canal carcinoma. J Laryngol Otol 2003;117(12):951–4.

44. Sasaki CT. Distant metastases from ear and temporal bone cancer. ORL J Otorhinolaryngol Relat Spec 2001;63(4):250–1.

45. Yin M, Ishikawa K, Honda K, et al. Analysis of 95 cases of squamous cell carcinoma of the external and middle ear. Auris Nasus Larynx 2006;33(3):251–7.

46. Rinaldo A, Ferlito A, Suarez C, et al. Nodal disease in temporal bone squamous carcinoma. Acta Otolaryngol 2005;125(1):5–8.

47. Zanoletti E, Danesi G. The problem of nodal disease in squamous cell carcinoma of the temporal bone. Acta Otolaryngol 2010;130(8):913–6.

48. Mantravadi AV, Marzo SJ, Leonetti JP, et al. Lateral temporal bone and parotid malignancy with facial nerve involvement. Otolaryngol Head Neck Surg 2011;144(3):395–401.

49. McGrew BM, Jackson CG, Redtfeldt RA. Lateral skull base malignancies. Neurosurg Focus 2002;12(5):e8.

50. Lawton MT, Spetzler RF. Internal carotid artery sacrifice for radical resection of skull base tumors. Skull Base Surg 1996;6(2):119–23.

51. Feiz-Erfan I, Han PP, Spetzler RF, et al. Salvage of advanced squamous cell carcinomas of the head and neck: internal carotid artery sacrifice and extracranial-intracranial revascularization. Neurosurg Focus 2003;14(3):e6.

52. Sekhar LN, Pomeranz S, Janecka IP, et al. Temporal bone neoplasms: a report on 20 surgically treated cases. J Neurosurg 1992;76(4):578–87.

53. Moffat DA, Grey P, Ballagh RH, et al. Extended temporal bone resection for squamous cell carcinoma. Otolaryngol Head Neck Surg 1997;116(6 Pt 1):617–23.

54. Moffat DA, Wagstaff SA, Hardy DG. The outcome of radical surgery and postoperative radiotherapy for squamous carcinoma of the temporal bone. Laryngoscope 2005;115(2):341–7.

55. Barrs DM. Temporal bone carcinoma. Otolaryngol Clin North Am 2001;34(6):1197–218, x.

56. Manolidis S, Pappas D Jr, Von Doersten P, et al. Temporal bone and lateral skull base malignancy: experience and results with 81 patients. Am J Otol 1998;19(Suppl 6):S1–15.

57. Kang HC, Wu HG, Lee JH, et al. Role of radiotherapy for squamous cell carcinoma of the external auditory canal and middle ear. J Korean Soc Ther Radiol Oncol 2009;27(4):173–80.

58. Leonetti JP, Marzo SJ. Malignancy of the temporal bone. Otolaryngol Clin North Am 2002;35(2):405–10.

59. Bibas AG, Ward V, Gleeson MJ. Squamous cell carcinoma of the temporal bone. J Laryngol Otol 2008;122(11):1156–61.

60. Ogawa K, Nakamura K, Hatano K, et al. Treatment and prognosis of squamous cell carcinoma of the external auditory canal and middle ear: a multi-institutional retrospective review of 87 patients. Int J Radiat Oncol Biol Phys 2007;68(5):1326–34.

61. Pfreundner L, Schwager K, Willner J, et al. Carcinoma of the external auditory canal and middle ear. Int J Radiat Oncol Biol Phys 1999;44(4):777–88.

62. Prabhu R, Hinerman RW, Indelicato DJ, et al. Squamous cell carcinoma of the external auditory canal: long-term clinical outcomes using surgery and external-beam radiotherapy. Am J Clin Oncol 2009;32(4):401–4.

63. Cooper JS, Pajak TF, Forastiere AA, et al. Postoperative concurrent radiotherapy and chemotherapy for high-risk squamous-cell carcinoma of the head and neck. N Engl J Med 2004;350(19):1937–44.

64. Bernier J, Domenge C, Ozsahin M, et al. Postoperative irradiation with or without concomitant chemotherapy for locally advanced head and neck cancer. N Engl J Med 2004;350(19):1945–52.

65. Bonner JA, Harari PM, Giralt J, et al. Radiotherapy plus cetuximab for squamous-cell carcinoma of the head and neck. N Engl J Med 2006;354(6):567–78.

66. Posner MR, Wirth LJ. Cetuximab and radiotherapy for head and neck cancer. N Engl J Med 2006;354(6):634–6.

67. Posner MR, Hershock DM, Blajman CR, et al. Cisplatin and fluorouracil alone or with docetaxel in head and neck cancer. N Engl J Med 2007;357(17):1705–15.

68. Vermorken JB, Remenar E, van Herpen C, et al. Cisplatin, fluorouracil, and docetaxel in unresectable head and neck cancer. N Engl J Med 2007;357(17):1695–704.

69. Nakagawa T, Kumamoto Y, Natori Y, et al. Squamous cell carcinoma of the external auditory canal and middle ear: an operation combined with preoperative chemoradiotherapy and a free surgical margin. Otol Neurotol 2006;27(2):242–8 [discussion: 249].

70. Shiga K, Ogawa T, Maki A, et al. Concomitant chemoradiotherapy as a standard treatment for squamous cell carcinoma of the temporal bone. Skull Base 2011;21(3):153–8.

71. Sugimoto H, Ito M, Yoshida S, et al. Concurrent superselective intra-arterial chemotherapy and radiotherapy for late-stage squamous cell carcinoma of the temporal bone. Ann Otol Rhinol Laryngol 2011;120(6):372–6.

72. Lewis JS. Temporal bone resection. Review of 100 cases. Arch Otolaryngol 1975;101(1):23–5.

73. Lewis JS. Surgical management of tumors of the middle ear and mastoid. J Laryngol Otol 1983;97(4):299–311.

74. Madsen AR, Gundgaard MG, Hoff CM, et al. Cancer of the external auditory canal and middle ear in Denmark from 1992 to 2001. Head Neck 2008;30(10):1332–8.

75. Gillespie MB, Francis HW, Chee N, et al. Squamous cell carcinoma of the temporal bone: a radiographic-pathologic correlation. Arch Otolaryngol Head Neck Surg 2001;127(7):803–7.

76. Chang CH, Shu MT, Lee JC, et al. Treatments and outcomes of malignant tumors of external auditory canal. Am J Otolaryngol 2009;30(1):44–8.

77. Kinney SE, Wood BG. Malignancies of the external ear canal and temporal bone: surgical techniques and results. Laryngoscope 1987;97(2):158–64.

78. Gidley PW, Thompson CR, Roberts DB, et al. The results of temporal bone surgery for advanced or recurrent tumors of the parotid gland. Laryngoscope 2011;121(8):1702–7.

79. Kunst H, Lavieille JP, Marres H. Squamous cell carcinoma of the temporal bone: results and management. Otol Neurotol 2008;29(4):549–52.

Craniofacial Reconstruction Following Oncologic Resection

Matthew M. Hanasono, MD[a],*,
Theresa M. Hofstede, BSc, DDS[b]

KEYWORDS

- Skull base surgery • Microvascular free flap • Facial nerve reconstruction • Prosthesis
- Osseointegrated implants

KEY POINTS

- The goals of craniofacial reconstruction following skull base surgery include creating a watertight dural seal, providing a barrier between the dura and the aerodigestive tract, supporting the orbit, and restoring facial appearance and function.
- Classifying skull base lesions into regions based on key anatomic structures helps to predict the reconstructive needs and outcomes.
- Repair and rehabilitation of the facial nerve, if resected, must be considered in the reconstructive approach.
- Prosthetic rehabilitation may be the most appropriate way of replacing resected facial structures such as the eye, nose, or ear, or may be used while awaiting autologous tissue reconstruction.

INTRODUCTION

Neoplasms involving the skull base are among the most challenging tumors to treat. The complex anatomy of the region makes resection difficult and places the patient at risk for major complications, such as cerebrospinal fluid (CSF) leak, meningitis, and osteomyelitis. Craniofacial reconstructions that minimize the risks for such complications as well as restore facial appearance and function have become a critical part of most skull base surgeries (**Box 1**). Although, historically, skull base resections were associated with poor outcomes, advances in reconstruction, which minimize complications, loss of function, and disfigurement, concomitant with advances in oncologic resection, radiation, chemotherapy, and diagnostic and interventional radiology, have substantially decreased the morbidity as well as increased the efficacy of skull base tumor treatment.

The objective of this article is to describe an algorithm for defects encountered following skull base resection, focusing primarily on microvascular free flap reconstruction. Although local flaps remain useful for a few specific indications, microvascular free flaps are now used for most skull base reconstructions.[1,2] Unlike local flaps, which are limited in reach and volume, free flaps permit virtually unlimited degrees of freedom in their placement and can be tailored precisely with respect to size and tissue type (eg, bone, muscle, adipose tissue, skin).[3,4] Techniques for treating facial nerve paralysis are also discussed because the facial nerve is frequently resected in skull base surgeries. Finally, prosthetic rehabilitation

Disclosures and conflicts of interest: Dr Hanasono, none; Dr Hofstede, none.
[a] Department of Plastic Surgery, The University of Texas MD Anderson Cancer Center, 1515 Holcombe Boulevard, Unit 443, Houston, TX 77030, USA; [b] Section of Dental Oncology, Department of Head and Neck Surgery, The University of Texas MD Anderson Cancer Center, 1515 Holcombe Boulevard, Unit 1445, Houston, TX 77030, USA
* Corresponding author.
E-mail address: mhanasono@mdanderson.org

Neurosurg Clin N Am 24 (2013) 111–124
http://dx.doi.org/10.1016/j.nec.2012.08.006
1042-3680/13/$ – see front matter © 2013 Elsevier Inc. All rights reserved.

of face, which allows restoration of delicate facial features in ways that may be more expedient, more straightforward, or, at times, even more aesthetic than reconstruction with autologous tissues, is addressed.

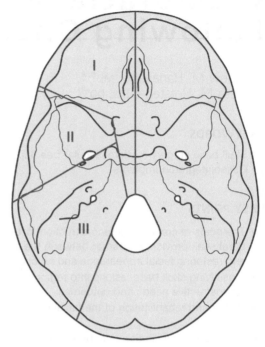

Fig. 1. Skull base regions.

CLASSIFICATION

Oncologic skull base defects can be broadly defined as those occurring from resection of tumors arising from or involving the floor of the anterior, middle, or posterior cranial fossae. These resections involve removal of cranial bone, with or without incision of the dura. The classification system described by Irish and colleagues[5] remains the most useful for describing skull base tumors because it communicates the general location of the defects and predicts the reconstructive challenges associated with a given region of the skull base (**Fig. 1**).

Briefly, region I involves defects from tumors arising from the orbits and sinuses, those extending into the anterior cranial fossae, and those originating in the clivus or extending as far posteriorly as the foramen magnum. Region II defects result from tumors originating from the lateral skull base, primarily the infratemporal and pterygopalatine fossae, which may extend into the middle cranial fossa. Region III defects are almost all associated with tumors arising from the ear, parotid, or temporal bone, and may extend into the middle or posterior cranial fossae.

REGION I

Region I resections may involve the central or lateral anterior cranial fossa, or both. Central region I tumors often originate from the ethmoid and sphenoid sinuses or the cribriform plate, as is the case with esthesioneuroblastomas. Tumors in region I are usually resected with an anterior craniofacial approach, resulting in a communication of the nasal cavity with the intracranial space. Skull base defects restricted to the upper nasal cavity can be reconstructed with a pericranial flap or a galea-frontalis flap, transposed to line the floor of the anterior cranial fossa.[5] Sizable defects that encompass the external nose, forehead, and/or orbit, are usually best reconstructed with a free flap.

Nasal reconstructions are usually addressed separately from the skull base. Such reconstructions are delicate, multistaged procedures using local flaps, such as the paramedian forehead flap, and auricular or costal cartilage grafts. Reconstruction is usually delayed for many months following the conclusion of adjuvant radiation therapy, if given, to avoid fibrosis and contracture of the reconstructed nose. Prostheses are another option for nasal reconstruction that often produce an even better aesthetic result than autologous tissues and do not require multiple operations (see later discussion).

Lateral region I tumors may arise from orbital or periorbital structures and frequently involve orbital exenteration or orbitomaxillectomy. In orbital exenterations that spare the medial and inferior orbital walls, a thin fasciocutaneous free flap, such as the radial forearm fasciocutaneous free flap, can resurface the orbit, and protect exposed dura and bone. If the patient desires an orbital prosthesis, reconstruction with thin flaps results in a concave orbital cavity that is suited to prosthetic retention.[6]

A temporalis muscle pedicled flap can also be used to resurface the orbital cavity. In such cases, it is often necessary to remove the lateral wall of the orbit to extend the reach of the flap.[1] One disadvantage of the temporalis muscle flap is that it usually leaves a noticeable hollowing in the temporal fossa. However, the donor site hollowing can often be addressed satisfactorily with autologous fat grafting performed as an outpatient elective secondary procedure.

In orbitomaxillectomies and orbital exenterations that result in communication with the nasal and sinus cavities, bulkier flaps, such as the anterolateral thigh (ALT) or rectus abdominis myocutaneous (RAM) free flaps, more reliably close orbital wall dehiscences (**Fig. 2**).[6] Both flaps have the advantage of being highly versatile with respect to including a variable amount of muscle (ie, the vastus lateralis muscle in the ALT free flap and the rectus abdominis muscle in the RAM free flap) to reach the volume needed. Conversely, both flaps can usually be harvested with minimal or no muscle and even thinned (primarily or during a secondary procedure) when less thickness is desired.[7,8]

In the authors' experience, it is usually preferable to include enough flap tissue for region I reconstructions so that all dehiscences are sealed to minimize the chances of a developing a sinonasal-cutaneous fistula. Such fistulae, although not dangerous to the patient, rarely, if ever, heal spontaneously due to the air pressures generated by nasal breathing and nose blowing. One drawback of filling the orbit with flap tissue is that prosthetic retention may be difficult and the prosthesis may protrude unnaturally due to the lack of a concave orbit.

REGION II

Region II extends from the petrous temporal bone to the posterior orbital wall and includes the infratemporal and pterygomaxillary fossae. Tumors that originate in this region include nasopharyngeal tumors, glomus jugulare tumors, meningiomas, and clival chordomas as well as parotid tumors that grow deeply and maxillary or even cheek neoplasms that spread posteriorly, usually via the maxillary division of the trigeminal nerve (V2).

Resection of region II tumors may involve an anterior transmaxillary approach.[2] When the skull base has been resected, leaving the dura exposed, the defect must be reconstructed to isolate the intracranial contents from the nasal cavity, ruling out prosthetic obturation as a potential method of

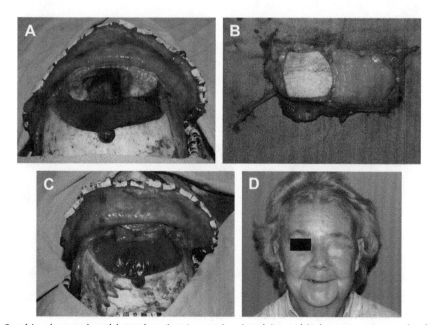

Fig. 2. (*A*) Combined central and lateral region I resection involving orbital exenteration and a frontal craniotomy, resulting in communication of the anterior cranial fossa with the orbital and sinonasal cavities. (*B*) Anterolateral thigh free flap designed to separate the intracranial cavity from the sinonasal and orbital cavities. (*C*) Flap inset. (*D*) Postoperative result.

reconstruction. Muscle or myocutaneous flaps are used to obliterate the maxillary cavity (**Fig. 3**).

The temporalis muscle may reach this area, but often does not provide adequate bulk to restore facial contour when the maxillary buttresses have been resected, especially in the face of radiation-associated atrophy. In such cases, a myocutaneous free flap, such as the ALT and RAM free flaps, are usually better choices. When there is no oral or cheek defect, the skin paddle of the free flap can be de-epithelialized and the entire flap buried. The muscle component usually provides an adequate seal against dural leaks.[1] The adipose component of the flap usually undergoes minimal atrophy, even following radiation, such that facial contours are maintained and adequate support of the skull base is achieved to prevent brain herniation.

Accurate reconstruction of the orbital floor is mandatory if included as part of the resection while sparing the globe.[8] Malposition of the orbital floor can result in enophthalmos, exophthalmos, or vertical dystopia (eyes at unequal heights). Most of what is known about orbital floor reconstruction comes from the trauma literature. Both alloplastic materials, such as titanium mesh or porous polyethylene, as well as autogenous grafts, such as calvarial or iliac crest bone grafts, have been successfully used. Autogenous grafts have the theoretic advantage of revascularization by the surrounding tissues, making them potentially more resistant to radiation-associated complications, such as infection or exposure. The authors' experience does not strongly support use of one material over another; however, well-vascularized tissue coverage of the entire implant or graft is mandatory, regardless of the material used, if postoperative radiation is planned. Care must also be taken not to impinge on the optic nerve during orbital floor reconstruction.

Some resections for tumors in region II are approached laterally instead of anteriorly. These resections require removal of several structures, including the parotid, posterior mandible, and posterolateral maxilla. For these defects, which may include both a cutaneous component and an intraoral component, the authors use the ALT and RAM free flaps to reconstruct the oral defect separately from the facial defect. These can be designed to include multiple skin paddles based on separate perforators. Good results with soft tissue reconstruction alone can be achieved for posterior mandibular defects.[9,10] Resections that encompass both regions I and II often involve orbitomaxillectomies and are reconstructed in an identical manner to those orbitomaxillectomies that only

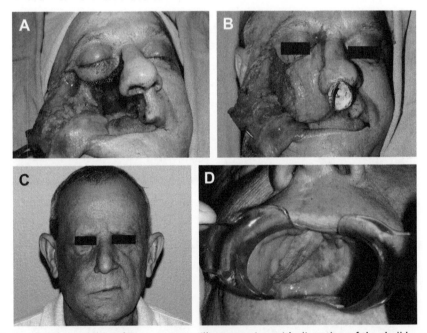

Fig. 3. (*A*) Region II defect resulting from a transmaxillary resection with dissection of the skull base around the foramen rotundum due to cancer spread along the maxillary division of the trigeminal nerve. The orbital floor has been reconstructed with titanium mesh. (*B*) An anterolateral thigh free flap, covering the skull base defect and separating the dura from the maxillary sinus, as well as supporting the titanium mesh implant. (*C*) Postoperative result. (*D*) Intraoral skin paddle used to reconstruct the palate.

involve region I, with a bulky free flap that fills both the orbit and the sinus cavities.

REGION III

Region III tumors include cutaneous tumors involving the external auditory canal, such as squamous and basal cell carcinomas, as well as parotid tumors and, occasionally, sarcomas that arise directly from the temporal bone. In region III, small defects are often amenable to reconstruction with the temporalis muscle flap, which lies within the operative field, provided that the blood supply, the anterior and posterior deep temporal branches of the internal maxillary artery, remains intact.[11] The radial forearm fasciocutaneous free flap can also be used for small superficial defects, such as those arising from a partial or total auriculectomy.[12,13]

The ALT and RAM free flaps work well in this region when a larger flap is needed (**Fig. 4**).[14,15] They are configured such that a muscle component to the flap fills the deep portion of the wound and the skin paddle resurfaces the cutaneous defect, if there is one. If there is no cutaneous defect, the skin paddle can be de-epithelialized and entirely buried as discussed for region II defects. Although latissimus dorsi muscle free flaps, covered by a split-thickness skin graft, is often used to reconstruct very large defects involving the scalp, ALT free flaps also have reliably closed very large defects. Reconstructions for defects that include both region II and III also tend to require larger, bulky free flaps, occasionally with two skin paddles if an oral cavity defect exists in addition to an external defect.[15]

The pectoralis major, trapezius, and even the latissimus dorsi myocutaneous pedicled flaps

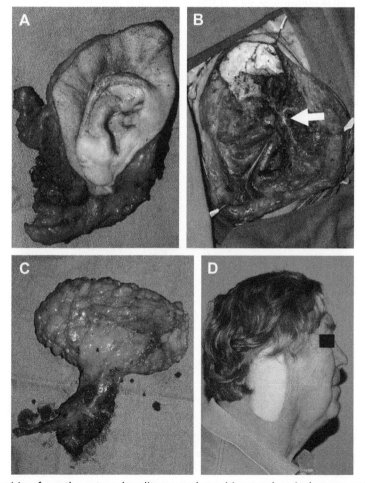

Fig. 4. (*A*) Tumor arising from the external auditory canal requiring total auriculectomy and lateral temporal bone resection. (*B*) Resulting region III defect. (*C*) Anterolateral thigh free flap designed as a myocutaneous free flap. The muscle component will go into the temporal bone defect, protecting the sigmoid sinus, and obliterating the eustachian tube orifice. (*D*) Postoperative result.

have also been used to reconstruct defects of region III. The authors restrict their use to modest defects only in patients who are not candidates for free flaps and in whom the temporalis muscle flap is unavailable or of inadequate size to perform the reconstruction. Pedicled flaps from the torso often have problems with reaching the superior most portion of the surgical defect. Even when they do reach, the closure is tight and postoperative fibrosis of the muscular pedicle usually restricts neck movement. When neck movement becomes restricted or there is an aesthetically unappealing bulkiness in the neck due to the mass of the muscular pedicle, a revision procedure to debulk the proximal flap can be performed 3 months after the initial surgery or 6 months following the conclusion of postoperative radiation, whichever is later.[2]

The external ear, if resected, is usually best reconstructed separately in a delayed manner if postoperative radiation is anticipated, as it is with nasal reconstruction. Prosthetic rehabilitation (see later discussion) for total auricular reconstruction is usually the mainstay in oncologic surgery due to the lack of thin, pliable cutaneous tissue to cover a cartilaginous framework carved from costochondral grafts or alloplasts such as porous polyethylene. Partial defects of the auricle can be reconstructed with local tissue flaps or incorporated into the design of a free flap used to close the skull base wound and eliminate dead space.

Our institutional treatment algorithm is summarized in **Fig. 5**. Microvascular free flaps are selected over regional flaps whenever vascularized tissue coverage is needed and regional flaps are not suitable due to limitations in size, reach, or reliability. Additionally, microvascular free flaps should be used in medically suitable candidates whenever such reconstruction holds promise for a better quality of life via improved function or aesthetic appearance than can be achieved with other techniques. Because placement of either a regional or a free flap may inhibit the ability to detect a local recurrence by physical examination, serial imaging is mandatory for disease surveillance.

With regard to recipient artery choice for microvascular free flaps, the facial and superficial temporal arteries are most commonly used in region I, the facial artery is most commonly used in region II, and the facial and distal external carotid arteries are most commonly used in region III, all based on proximity to the defect. Similar to recipient artery choice, the facial and superficial temporal veins are most commonly used in region I. In regions II and III, the facial and internal jugular

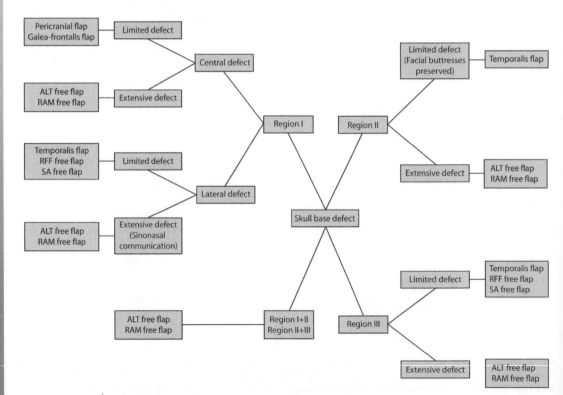

Fig. 5. Institutional algorithm for oncologic skull base reconstruction.

veins are most commonly used. The transverse cervical artery and vein are occasionally useful as recipient vessels in region III when the external carotid artery and internal jugular vein, or their branches, are not available.

FACIAL NERVE

Malignancies that involve the skull base, particularly those that arise from the parotid gland or the temporal bone, may invade the facial nerve. Additionally, surgeries to remove skull base tumors may also put the facial nerve at risk. Facial nerve sacrifice usually causes marked deformity and may significantly affect a patient's quality of life. Loss of facial nerve function not only entails a cosmetic defect but also a functional one, including difficulty with eye closure, nasal breathing, and oral competence, as well as a tendency to bite the buccal and upper lip mucosa. Although facial nerve repair is feasible in many cases, some surgeons are reluctant to consider it because of a misconception that nerve regeneration is unlikely, specifically in patients with preoperative dysfunction or advanced age, or when postoperative radiation therapy is planned.

Results of facial nerve repair following treatment of malignancy have been documented in a few recent studies.[2,16,17] The authors have observed at least some facial nerve recovery in most patients who underwent cable nerve graft repair following a skull base resection that entailed nerve division.[2] Return of function was noted to occur at a mean time of 7.7 months postoperatively, although regeneration was noted as late as 21.4 months after repair. Recovery was observed even in patients with prior weakness or paralysis, postoperative radiation, and advanced age, although less predictably than in patients without these risk factors. The authors did not perform any repairs in patients with complete paralysis of greater than 12 months duration because of motor endplate degeneration that occurs in the face of long-standing paralysis.

Iseli and colleagues[16] reported at least some facial nerve recovery at a median time of 6.2 months postoperatively in 97% of their series of 33 patients who underwent facial nerve grafting following skull base resection, although their patient population contained a different mix of follow-up time, preoperative function, age, and radiation history. Taken together, results from these studies argue for performing facial nerve repair in all patients whenever feasible regardless of the presence of risk factors for poor reinnervation, based on the assumption that even some recovery results in improved function and appearance. An inability to locate the proximal and distal ends of the facial nerve or a long period of facial paralysis before surgery (>12 months) are the main contraindications to performing nerve repair or grafting. Before surgery, patients should be counseled about potential nonrecovery or incomplete recovery of facial nerve function, as well as synkinesis.

Besides nerve repair, static facial nerve rehabilitative procedures can also be of great help to patients. Static procedures include: browlift, upper eyelid gold weight placement, lateral canthoplasty, lateral tarsorrhaphy, and static lower facial reanimation with a fascial sling. Patients should be evaluated preoperatively and at subsequent follow-up appointments for brow ptosis, incomplete eye closure, ectropion, oral incompetence, and facial asymmetry. Based on these findings, static procedures are then performed accordingly (**Table 1**).

Several types of browlifts have been described including direct, midforehead, coronal, and endoscopic. Most patients with unilateral brow dysfunction are best served with a direct browlift, involving an excision of skin along the superior border of the eyebrow and fixation of the brow to the forehead periosteum. The goals of the browlift are to restore symmetry in repose with the

Table 1
Static procedures for loss of facial nerve function

Nerve Deficit	Problem	Recommended Procedure
Temporal branch	Brow ptosis	Direct browlift
Zygomatic branches	Corneal exposure	Upper eyelid gold weight placement, possible lateral tarsorrhaphy
Zygomatic branches	Ectropion	Lateral canthoplasty, possible lower lid fascial sling
Buccal branches	Oral incompetence, nasal obstruction, facial asymmetry	Fascial sling, possible unilateral or differential facelift

contralateral (normal) side and to prevent obstruction of the superior visual field. In youth, a boy's brow usually rests at the level of the superior orbital rim, while the lateral portion of a girl's brow rests slightly above, peaking in line with the lateral limbus of the eye. When the brows demonstrate significant ptosis such that a unilateral symmetrizing procedure still results in superior visual field obstruction, a bilateral browlift, in which both brows are restored to a youthful position, might be considered. A bilateral endoscopic or coronal browlift might be aesthetically more favorable in this situation.

The eyelids serve to protect the eye as well as to direct tears into the tear ducts. Although the oculomotor nerve (III) is responsible for eye opening and is usually preserved in most skull base surgeries (at least those that preserve the orbit), the facial nerve is responsible for eye closure. Gold weights are the mainstay of methods for improving upper lid closure, although springs and platinum weights are also used by some surgeons. Standard weights range from 0.6 g to 1.8 g. Sizing weights, which are placed on the upper lid with adhesives in the office, are used to help select the appropriate weight. Most patients are adequately corrected with a 1.0 g weight in the authors' experience, so we use this as a starting point.

Gold weights are placed into a precise pocket made on top of the tarsal plate of the upper eyelid, though a supratarsal crease incision.[18] There are holes in the weight that allow fixation with suture to the perichondrium of the tarsal plate (we use 7-0 polypropylene [Prolene] for fixation). The supratarsal incision is closed with absorbable suture, such as 6-0 fast-absorbing gut. All patients with facial nerve sacrifice must be counseled regarding eye protection and lubrication with artificial tears and more viscous lubricants, particularly at night. Signs or symptoms of exposure keratitis should be referred to an ophthalmologist promptly.

A lateral canthoplasty, also known as a tarsal strip procedure, tightens the lower lid to correct ectropion. In this procedure, the lateral tarsus is denuded and suspended to the upper, inner lateral orbital periosteum. Such a procedure may not be needed in younger patients with good skin elasticity. A lateral tarsorrhaphy can complement a gold weight and a lateral canthoplasty to help narrow the eyelid aperture and prevent desiccation of the cornea. Several millimeters of the lateral upper and lower lid margin are de-epithelialized and a buried suture is placed to create an adhesion. Care is taken to make sure the suture knot does not abrade the eye. Older patients, especially those with some degree of preexisting senile ectropion, may be inadequately corrected even with a lateral canthoplasty combined with a lateral tarsorrhaphy. In such patients, the medial lower lid also needs to be supported. A canthal sling created by suspending a fascia lata graft from the medial canthus to the lateral canthus can be used to address medial and residual lateral lagophthalmos.

Lower face fascial slings are static procedures used to prevent drooping of the cheek, which is not only aesthetically unpleasing but may also interfere with nasal breathing and oral competence. Patients with facial paralysis frequently complain of drooling, biting of the cheek mucosa, and ptosis of the upper lip affecting speech. Fascial slings are typically created using an autologous tensor fascia lata graft.[19] A single fascia lata graft split distally into multiple units or several independent grafts can be used to suspend the nasal ala, upper lip, and oral commissure to the zygomatic periosteum in the direction of muscular pull that mimics the contralateral zygomaticus muscles. The sling is tunneled between these points in a subcutaneous plane. Overcorrection is desirable because rapid descent of the fascial suspension is the norm following this procedure. Most surgeons recommend that the upper canine should be visible following correct tension setting of the graft. The fascial sling can usually be retightened if correction becomes inadequate over time.

Static facial nerve rehabilitative procedures can be performed immediately following the resection in conjunction with flap reconstruction or can be delayed and performed secondarily. However, when paralysis is anticipated, due to either preoperative paralysis or sacrifice of the facial nerve during surgery, immediate rehabilitation has the advantage of sparing the patient some of the morbidity of facial paralysis, especially during and immediately after adjuvant therapy when further surgery may be risky. Rose[19] and Deleyiannis and colleagues[20] have shown that facial nerve recovery is not prevented by facial paralysis rehabilitative procedures performed at the time of the initial surgery and think static procedures complement nerve repair. Golio and colleagues[21] also did not find a higher rate of complications nor an effect on symptomatic improvement in eye exposure in patients who had early periocular surgeries for facial nerve rehabilitation, before radiation therapy was administered, compared with patients who had the same procedures in a delayed setting. **Fig. 6** shows a patient who underwent static rehabilitative procedures simultaneously with facial nerve grafting and soft tissue free flap reconstruction.

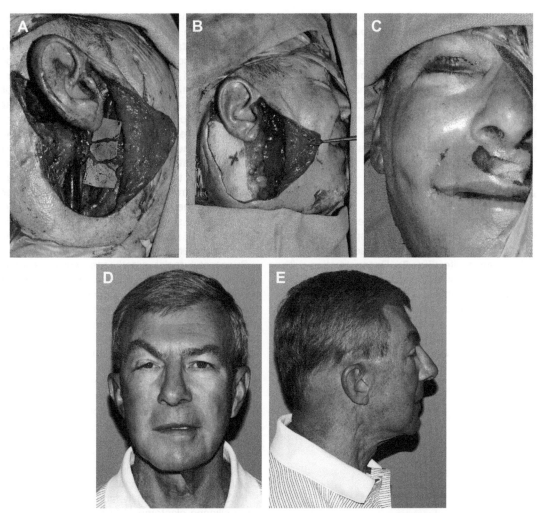

Fig. 6. (*A*) Facial nerve grafting following removal of a parotid malignancy. (*B*) Reconstruction of a region III defect with an anterolateral thigh free flap. (*C*) Placement of a fascial sling for static facial reanimation. (*D*, *E*) postoperative result showing reasonable facial symmetry at rest. An upper eyelid gold weight has been placed and a direct browlift has been performed.

In cases where the degree of dysfunction is not known preoperatively, the options are to perform static facial nerve rehabilitative surgery as a secondary procedure, allowing time to assess the degree of asymmetry before proceeding, or to perform the surgeries in the immediate setting, estimating the degree of correction needed. Although the former would seem logical, for practical purposes, it is often less morbid for the patient to undergo static procedures at the time of resection, to spare them some of the symptoms of facial paralysis, particularly if they must wait many months while they undergo and recover from adjuvant therapy before another surgery is possible. Timing of static procedures must, of course, be individualized to the patient and based on the expectations for nerve recovery as well as

the ability to undergo multiple operations versus a single longer operation.

For example, because many patients can develop exposure keratitis due to incomplete eye closure, a 1.0 g gold upper eyelid weight is placed at the time of surgical resection when the facial nerve has been divided. Adjustments can usually be deferred until after radiation and most patients can tolerate changing implants in the office, under local anesthesia. Browlifts are performed with the goal of achieving symmetry with the other side in repose. Fascial slings are usually set to a standard degree of overcorrection in all patients. Placement of fascial slings, in particular, can be hazardous when performed as a delayed procedure if there is a chance of injuring recovering facial nerve grafts, as well as poorly healing radiated cheek skin. Lateral canthoplasties are performed such that the lower lid is raised to a youthful position, eliminating all ectropion. If satisfactory recovery does occur following a nerve repair, some static procedures can be reversed. Specifically, gold weights can be removed, tarsorrhaphies can be lysed, and fascial slings can be divided or removed. Other procedures, such as browlifts and canthoplasties, can usually be left alone or, if anything, contralateral procedures may be indicated, particularly in the aged.

PROSTHETIC RESTORATION

Surgical ablation of facial structures, such as the eyes, ears, and nose, are usually especially devastating for a patient's appearance, self-confidence, and quality of life (**Fig. 7**). Reconstruction with autologous tissue is desirable; however, it may not be an attainable goal. The limitations of surgical reconstruction may include inadequate adjacent tissue, poor color, texture, and/or contour match of flap tissue to facial tissue, the need for multiple surgeries to achieve a desirable

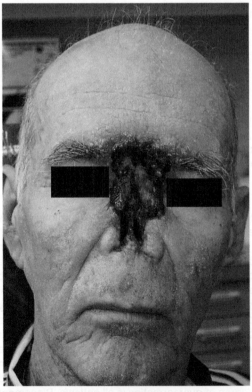

Fig. 7. Postsurgical near total rhinectomy shows a large defect that is not easily amenable to surgical reconstruction. This disfigurement affects a patient's self-confidence and ability to interact socially. Prosthetic rehabilitation can restore confidence and quality of life.

result, contraindications to surgery due to comorbidities of the patient, and an inability to meet patient expectations. Autologous reconstruction may also be contraindicated due to the need for surveillance of the surgical site for tumor recurrence or relatively contraindicated because of a high chance of recurrence, making it likely that further resection may be required. In these situations, a prosthesis may be custom made by maxillofacial prosthodontists and anaplastologists to closely replicate the presurgical contour, color, and texture of the ablated structure.[22] Rehabilitation with a maxillofacial prosthesis may offer a highly aesthetic and predictable alternative to reconstructive surgery or act as a temporary solution for those patients who are awaiting reconstructive surgery.

Successful facial prostheses require a well-healed defect, without mobile or compressible underlying tissue, exposed bone, or bulky convex flaps. Excessively mobile tissue can compromise prosthesis retention. During surgical ablation, any exposed bone should be smoothed and then overlaid with a split thickness skin graft because it provides a nonmobile, durable tissue site, which is ideal for prosthesis placement (**Fig. 8**). If skin graft take is expected to be poor (eg, over radiated bone) and a flap is required for bone coverage, then the flap will often need to be thinned primarily or secondarily before prosthesis placement.[22] Bulky flaps can occupy the space required for the prosthesis, interfering with its retention or causing it to protrude unnaturally from the face.

Prostheses are typically fabricated from a platinum silicone elastomer that provides good form and durability as well as flexibility. With normal use, the silicone can move with the surrounding tissue without detaching. This material can be intrinsically and extrinsically colored and textured to replicate skin features. The longevity of silicone, however, is limited because it is subject to discoloration, degradation, and edge tearing with daily use. Silicone facial prostheses typically require replacement annually. Acrylic resins can be used in combination in the fabrication of facial prostheses. This rigid plastic can provide a substructure that supports or connects to the silicone elastomer portion of the prosthesis. The acrylic resin is also used to construct the ocular (eye globe) of the orbital prosthetic. Acrylic resin is rarely used to fabricate the entire prosthesis because it lacks the flexibility to move with the underlying tissue, which helps with retention.[23] Prostheses can also be made with a polyurethane liner on the tissue-bearing surface to improve tear resistance of the edges and aid in inhibiting microbial growth inherent to silicone.[24]

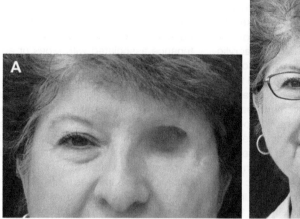
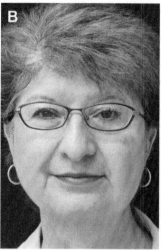

Fig. 8. Postsurgical orbital exenteration reveals large defect. Prosthetic rehabilitation of orbital defects provides superior esthetics, unattainable by surgical reconstruction. (*A*) A split-thickness skin graft lines the bony orbital defect and provides a durable base for prosthesis placement. (*B*) Completed orbital prosthesis has superior esthetics by replicating the presurgical contour, color, and texture. Patients are encouraged to wear glasses to protect their functioning eye.

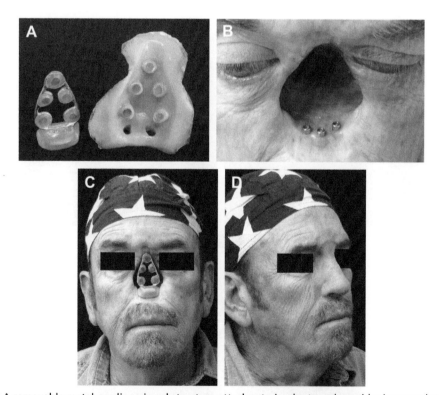

Fig. 9. (*A*) A removable metal-acrylic resin substructure attaches to implants and provides improved stability and retention of the prosthetic. The embedded magnets correspond to countermagnets on the tissue surface of the nasal prosthetic and aid in its orientation. (*B*) Endosteal implants in the maxillary alveolar bone with the prosthetic abutments extending into the nasal cavity. (*C*) The removable metal-acrylic resin substructure attaches to implants in the inferior nasal cavity. (*D*) Nasal prosthetic in position. Adhesives and/or tape are not necessary for retention.

Orbital, auricular, and nasal prostheses are the most common prostheses used for in patients with head and neck cancer. These prostheses are designed to be removable and are fixed to the underlying tissues with one or more of the following: glue, tape, magnets (built into acrylic substructures), tissue undercuts, and endosteal implants. Medical-grade adhesives can hold facial prostheses for up to 10 hours; however, retention may be affected by excessive movement, perspiration, and environmental conditions.[25] Double-sided tapes provide good prosthetic retention and ease of use, but may damage the thin edges of the prosthesis and cause tissue irritation with repeated placement and removal. An acrylic resin substructure can be placed into nonmobile undercuts of the surgical defect and retain the facial prosthesis with matching samarium cobalt magnets in both segments of the prostheses.[26] Osseointegrated craniofacial implants provide a direct bond to the surrounding bone and can offer excellent prosthesis retention (**Fig. 9**).[27-32] Various transcutaneous attachments (abutments) are available that screw into the implant and provide many methods for prosthesis connection. Compared with other methods of retention, osseointegrated implants have improved retention and stability, reduce skin irritation, enhance patient comfort and confidence, reduce the maintenance associated with tapes or adhesives, and increase prosthesis longevity.[33,34]

Facial prostheses are created by making an accurate impression of the defect and its surrounding tissue. If a substructure or implants are present, orientation of those elements are registered in the impression. Dental stone is poured into the intaglio surface of the impression to obtain the patient cast or model. A thin sheet of tin foil is burnished onto the stone and then the missing facial structure is sculpted with wax or modeling clay. The patient then "tries on" the sculpting multiple times to assess its form, adaptation, and orientation. Once complete, the sculpting is processed by encasing it in a stone mold, removing the wax or clay, and then replacing the void in the mold with skin colored silicone. Once the silicone has cured, the facial prosthesis is fitted to the patient's defect and then extrinsically

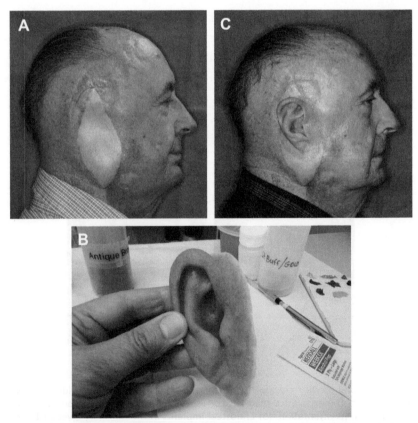

Fig. 10. (*A*) Auricular defect that has been reconstructed with a soft tissue flap. (*B*) This auricular prosthetic must be retained with medical adhesive or double-sided tape. (*C*) Facial prostheses are custom made for each patient to optimize adaptation, color, and skin texture.

colored to match the unique skin tones and textures using silicone adhesive and pigments (**Fig. 10**).

SUMMARY

Skull base reconstruction has evolved greatly, facilitating surgical resection by reducing the rate of major complications such as dural exposure, pneumocephalus, and CSF leakage. Patient morbidity is further reduced by soft tissue free flap reconstruction to restore the contours of the patient's face, as well as facial nerve reconstruction and rehabilitation procedures in cases in which the nerve is involved or must be sacrificed to achieve an oncologically sound tumor removal. Prosthetic rehabilitation, sometimes combined with osseointegrated titanium implants for stable fixation, helps to restore fine facial features such as the nose, eyes, and ears, particularly in cases in which autologous tissue reconstruction is not feasible or not desired by the patient.

REFERENCES

1. Chang DW, Langstein HN, Gupta A, et al. Reconstructive management of cranial base defects after tumor ablation. Plast Reconstr Surg 2001;107: 1346–55.

2. Hanasono MM, Silva AK, Skoracki RJ, et al. Skull base reconstruction: an updated approach. Plast Reconstr Surg 2011;128:675–86.

3. Neligan PC, Mulholland S, Irish J, et al. Flap selection in cranial base reconstruction. Plast Reconstr Surg 1996;98:1159–66.

4. Califano J, Cordeiro PG, Disa JJ, et al. Anterior cranial base reconstruction using free tissue transfer: changing tends. Head Neck 2003;25:89–96.

5. Irish J, Gullane PJ, Gentili F, et al. Tumors of the skull base: outcome and survival analysis of 77 cases. Head Neck 1994;16:3–10.

6. Hanasono MM, Lee JC, Yang JS, et al. An algorithmic approach to reconstructive surgery and prosthetic rehabilitation after orbital exenteration. Plast Reconstr Surg 2009;123:98–105.

7. Amin A, Rifaat M, Civantos F, et al. Free anterolateral thigh flap for reconstruction of major craniofacial defects. J Reconstr Microsurg 2006;22:97–104.

8. Chiu ES, Kraus D, Bui DT, et al. Anterior and middle cranial fossa skull base reconstruction using microvascular free tissue techniques. Ann Plast Surg 2008;60:514–20.

9. Mosahebi A, Chaudhry A, McCarthy CM, et al. Reconstruction of extensive composite posterolateral mandibular defects using nonosseous free tissue transfer. Plast Reconstr Surg 2009;124:1571–7.

10. Hanasono MM, Zevallos JP, Skoracki RJ, et al. A prospective analysis of bony versus soft-tissue reconstruction for posterior mandibular defects. Plast Reconstr Surg 2010;125:1413–21.

11. Hanasono MM, Utley DS, Good RL. The temporalis muscle flap for reconstruction after head and neck oncologic surgery. Laryngoscope 2001;111:1719–25.

12. Rosenthal EL, King K, McGrew BM, et al. Evolution of a paradigm for free tissue transfer reconstruction of lateral temporal bone defects. Head Neck 2008; 30:589–94.

13. Disa JJ, Rodriguez VM, Cordeiro PG. Reconstruction of lateral skull base oncological defects: the role of free tissue transfer. Ann Plast Surg 1998;41: 633–9.

14. Hanasono MM, Sacks JM, Goel N, et al. The anterolateral thigh free flap for skull base reconstruction. Otolaryngol Head Neck Surg 2009;140:855–60.

15. Moncrieff MD, Hamilton SA, Lamberty GH, et al. Reconstructive options after temporal bone resection for squamous cell carcinoma. J Plast Reconstr Aesthet Surg 2007;60:607–14.

16. Malata CM, Terhani H, Kumiponjera D, et al. Use of anterolateral thigh and lateral arm fasciocutaneous free flaps in lateral skull base reconstruction. Ann Plast Surg 2006;57:169–75.

17. Iseli TA, Harris G, Dean NR, et al. Outcomes of static and dynamic facial nerve repair in head and neck cancer. Laryngoscope 2010;120:478–83.

18. Gidley PW, Herrera SJ, Hanasono MM, et al. The impact of radiotherapy on facial nerve repair. Laryngoscope 2010;120:1985–9.

19. Rose EH. Autogenous fascia lata grafts: clinical applications in reanimation of the totally or partially paralyzed face. Plast Reconstr Surg 2005;116:20–32.

20. Deleyiannis FW, Askari M, Schmidt KL, et al. Muscle activity in the partially paralyzed face after placement of a fascial sling: a preliminary report. Ann Plast Surg 2005;55:449–55.

21. Golio D, De Matelaere S, Anderson J, et al. Outcomes of periocular reconstruction for facial nerve paralysis in cancer patients. Plast Reconstr Surg 2007;119:1233–7.

22. Lemon JC, Chambers MS, Martin JW. Prosthetic rehabilitation of patients with advanced nonmelanoma skin cancer. Clin Plast Surg 1997;24(4):797–815.

23. Heller HL, McKinstry RE. Facial materials. In: McKinstry RE, editor. Fundamentals of facial prosthetics. Arlington (TX): ABI Professional Publications; 1995. p. 84–5.

24. Udagama A. Urethane-lined silicone facial prostheses. J Prosthet Dent 1987;58(3):351–4.

25. Lemon JC, Chambers MS. Conventional methods of retention of facial prostheses. In: Beumer J, Zlotolow I, Esposito S, editors. Proceedings of the 1st International Congress on Maxillofacial Prosthetics. Memorial Sloan-Kettering Cancer Center 1995;1:116–9.

26. Mekayarajjananonth T, Huband ML, Guerra LR. Clear acrylic resin device for orientation and placement of a small facial prosthesis. J Prosthet Dent 2000; 83(6):656–9.

27. Miles BA, Sinn DP, Gion GG. Experience with cranial implant-based prosthetic reconstruction. J Craniofac Surg 2006;17(5):889–97.

28. Tjellstrom A. Osseointegrated implants for replacement of absent or defective ears. Clin Plast Surg 1990;17(2):355–66.

29. Tolman DE, Taylor PF. Bone-anchored craniofacial prosthesis study: irradiated patients. Int J Oral Maxillofac Implants 1996;11(5):612–9.

30. Wolfaardt JF, Wilkes GH, Parel SM, et al. Craniofacial osseointegration: the Canadian experience. Int J Oral Maxillofac Implants 1993;8(2):197–204.

31. Parel SM, Tjellstrom A. The United States and Swedish experience with osseointegration and facial prostheses. Int J Oral Maxillofac Implants 1991;6(1): 75–9.

32. Tolman DE, Taylor PF. Bone-anchored craniofacial prosthesis study. Int J Oral Maxillofac Implants 1996;11(2):159–68.

33. Beumer J, Marunick MT, Esposito SJ. In: Beumer J, Marunick MT, Esposito SJ, editors. Maxillofacial rehabilitation: rehabilitation of facial defects. Chicago: Quintessence Publishing Co, Inc; 2011. p. 285.

34. Jacobsson M, Tjellstrom A, Fine L, et al. An evaluation of auricular prosthesis using osseointegrated implants. Clin Otolaryngol Allied Sci 1992;17(6): 482–6.

Radiotherapy for Malignant Tumors of the Skull Base

Julian Johnson, MD, Igor J. Barani, MD*

KEYWORDS

- Linear accelerator • Gamma Knife • CyberKnife • Stereotactic • Skull base tumors

KEY POINTS

- Skull base tumors are a diverse group. They are often treated with adjuvant or definitive radiation for local control. This treatment concept arises from the difficulty of achieving aggressive gross total resections.
- Radiation therapy is a broad field, with many different treatment modalities, most of which are applicable to the skull base.
- Radiosurgery can be applied to smaller lesions if they are sufficiently far away from critical structures. Radiosurgery results in higher dose delivered to a tumor and structures very near to the prescription isodose line, with a rapid decline in radiation with distance.
- Conventional fractionation may be superior to radiosurgery in some cases. Generally, these are larger tumors interdigitated with a normal tissue, the radiotolerance of which exceeds that of the radiation dose needed to control a tumor.
- Conventional fractionation offers increasing conformality as a result of evolving treatment planning technology and beam arrangements, including three-dimensional conformal radiotherapy and intensity modulated radiation therapy.
- Proton beam radiotherapy offers unique advantages and is particularly useful in pediatric tumors and large tumors, which require more conformality than photon treatment plans may offer.

GENERATING THERAPEUTIC RADIATION

It is useful to be familiar with the scale of radiation under discussion. **Table 1** outlines radiation doses delivered in typical diagnostic and therapeutic procedures compared with common nonmedical radiation exposures.

When describing radiation doses, radiation oncologists use gray as the unit of choice. Proton doses are often expressed in Cobalt-Gray-Equivalents (CGE). Gray is a measurement of energy absorbed by tissue (joules per kilogram of tissue). Radiation safety typically uses units such as the sievert. The sievert expresses gray (absorbed dose) adjusted with a known constant, Q, which depends on the type of radiation in question. Protons, photons, and α particles each have different Q factors. The curie is a measurement that expresses radioactivity of a source before reaching a tissue. The curie is medically relevant when radioactive sources are used in brachytherapy. A detailed explanation of different means of measuring radiation is beyond the scope of this article.

Photons are the most commonly used therapeutic particle. High-energy electrons guided by a powerful magnet are directed toward a tungsten

Disclosures: Julian Johnson: None.
Conflict of Interest: Julian Johnson: None.
Department of Radiation Oncology, University of California, San Francisco, 505 Parnassus Avenue, Room L08, San Francisco, CA 94143-0226, USA
* Corresponding author.
E-mail address: Barani@radonc.ucsf.edu

Neurosurg Clin N Am 24 (2013) 125–135
http://dx.doi.org/10.1016/j.nec.2012.08.011
1042-3680/13/$ – see front matter © 2013 Elsevier Inc. All rights reserved.

Table 1
Radiation doses delivered in typical diagnostic and therapeutic procedures compared with common nonmedical radiation exposures. The University of California San Francisco and many others now require an accurate documentation in the medical record of radiation dose delivered during diagnostic procedures

Flight from LA to NY: 0.015 mSv
Dental X-ray: 0.09 mSv
Chest X-ray: 0.1 mSv
Mammogram: 0.7 mSv
Chest CT scan (low-dose): 1.5 mSv
Background Radiation: 6.2 mSv/year
Chest CT scan: 7 mSv
Abdominal CT scan: 10 mSv
Therapeutic Radiation (whole-brain): 30,000 mSv (30 Gy)
Therapeutic Radiation (brain tumor only): 50,000-60,000 mSv (50-60 Gy)

Where 1 Gy = 1000 mSv. Sievert is a measure of radiation effects adjusted for the type of radiation.

---

target. When the electrons strike the target, photons are generated via either the photoelectric or Compton effect, depending on the energy of the incident electron. Linear accelerators achieve this effect on a massive scale. Photons and γ rays are biologically and physically equivalent. Photons (or X-rays) are man-made whereas Gamma rays are generated by natural decay of a radioisotope. Both protons and γ rays can be used in the treatment of skull base tumors.

Protons are typically generated via a cyclotron. Only a few centers in the United States have proton machines, but the number of centers is rapidly increasing. Protons differ from photons in their dose distribution. The proton beam deposits maximum dose at a certain tissue depth determined by its energy, and then dose decreases precipitously, so-called "Bragg Peak" phenomenon.[1] Its use has been favored for pediatric tumors because of the theoretic lower risk of radiation exposure to nontarget tissues.

THE EFFECTS OF RADIATION

A detailed discussion about the manner in which ionizing radiation interacts with living cells is beyond the scope of this article. For the practicing physician or surgeon, it suffices to know that ionizing radiation exerts antitumor properties via a variety of potential effects on DNA. Direct radiation damage to DNA is probably less important. The most accepted primary cause of cell death is the double strand break, which triggers the apoptotic pathway. DNA suffers double strand breaks after interacting with free radicals, which are in turn generated by radiation effects on oxygen and water.

Given the importance of the presence of oxygen, more oxygenated cells in theory suffer greater radiation-induced damage. Fractionation allows tumors to reoxygenate, thereby fueling the DNA damaging process.

Fractionated external beam radiation therapy (EBRT) exploits the decreased ability of malignant cells to repair sublethal DNA damage. With each fraction, a new portion of abnormal cells reach a damage threshold. Although normal tissue repairs the damage more effectively, a greater portion of abnormal cells undergo cell death. Therefore it is possible to include normal tissue within a treatment field without completely destroying it. Even if tissues do not reach a lethal threshold, significant radiation damage may impair cellular function. The ability of normal tissues to recover from radiation injury varies by tissue type. Also, tissue dose tolerances vary when single high doses are given compared with fractionated radiotherapy (RT). For example, the optic chiasm does not seem to sustain clinically relevant damage if total fractionated dose is less than 50–54 Gy versus 8 Gy for single dose (**Fig. 1**). This is a particularly critical concept in the skull base, to which we return later in this article.

Target cells that do not reach lethal threshold with initial fractions accumulate more damage as they seek to replicate their DNA during mitosis. Tumors with a low mitotic fraction, number of cells undergoing active mitosis from a total tumor cell population, may experience a lesser response to radiation,[2] Many skull base tumors are in this category with characteristically low mitotic activity, such as meningiomas and schwannomas. Tumor control for these tumors is often defined as lack of growth rather than diminished size.

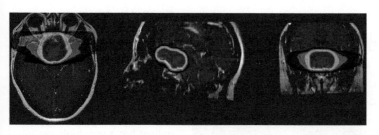

Fig. 1. Intensity modulated radiation therapy plan for a patient being treated for a WHO grade I meningioma that was resected 3 years before coming to our clinic. She presented with diplopia, headaches, and right lateral gaze palsy. Notice that the maximum radiation dose is focused around the tumor and a smaller, but not negligible, amount of radiation is delivered to surrounding structures. The red area represents the 95% isodose line. The other colors represent a gradient down to the 45% isodose line, which is in purple.

Radiosurgery uses very high doses of radiation, obliterating tumors and often inducing necrotic cell death. The entire target area receives 1 to 5 high, supralethal doses of radiation. These are often called ablative treatments because a greater portion of cells are directly destroyed by radiation rather than accumulating damage over time. The biological mechanisms underlying radiosurgical treatments are not well understood. A single fraction radiosurgery treatment may range from 10 to 80 Gy, whereas a typical fraction in conventionally fractionated RT is 1.8 to 2 Gy.

Often an increase in size may be observed after radiosurgery because of inflammatory reactions to necrotic tissue.[3] For example, Kollova and colleagues[4] observed perilesional edema in 15% of patients treated with stereotactic radiosurgery (SRS) for meningiomas. Once the necrotic tissue is cleared, tumors treated with SRS should decrease in size.

A BRIEF INTRODUCTION TO DELIVERY SYSTEM

With SRS of the skull base, it is critical to spare normal tissues in the immediate vicinity of the target in order not to cause normal tissue injury; therefore, tumors that encase functional structures are often not suitable for radiosurgical treatments. Radiosurgery is ideal for small targets (typically less than 2–3 cm), When targets are larger, the dose falloff with radiosurgery is less steep, the dose within the target less homogeneous, and the surrounding tissue exposed to significant levels of radiation increases. Radiosurgery can be accomplished with photons, γ rays, or protons. Linear accelerator based radiosurgery is performed with CyberKnife or a modified linear accelerator. Gamma Knife uses a Cobalt-60 source. There has been much debate about the merits of one SRS system over the other, but generally they are applied similar clinical situations Some institutions favor use of one radiosurgical modality over another despite absence of robust clinical data to justify such decisions. Most often, the use

and type of radiosurgical modality is governed by its availability. SRS is also accomplished with protons as well (**Fig. 2**).

Conventional radiation therapy delivered with linear accelerators is more widely available than SRS. Such treatments are ideal for larger targets not amenable to radiosurgery. EBRT is less conformal than radiosurgery and generally uses fewer beams. Each beam accounts for a higher portion of the total target dose, so exposure to surrounding tissues is inevitable (see **Fig. 1**).

All radiation treatments rely on strict, reproducible patient positioning and high-quality image guidance. The term "stereotactic" refers to the use of a three-dimensional coordinate space to which patient's anatomy and treatments are registered. Patient immobilization is therefore stricter for radiosurgery plans because high-doses of radiation are applied and the error is not distributed over many fractions. Patients being treated with Gamma Knife are immobilized with a metal frame affixed to the head. CyberKnife and EBRT treatments may be delivered with the patient's head immobilized using a custom-fitted thermoplastic mask that is used in conjuction with image-based corrections for deviations in patient position. New immobilization techniques are constantly evolving.

High-quality images are critical to radiation delivery. Obtaining images during treatment, the CyberKnife can automatically verify patient positioning in real time before delivering radiation. Conventional linear accelerators use cone beam computed tomography (CBCT) devices mounted on the linear accelerator to verify daily position with the images used to plan treatment. In the skull base, magnetic resonance imaging (MRI) scans fused with CT scans are increasingly used for planning purposes.

Brachytherapy is the use of a radioactive source isotope implanted into a patient (internal radiation) for dose delivery via catheters, seeds, or plaques. These sources are typically designed to have a rapid decline in dose delivered as a function of distance. They are particularly useful when it is necessary to deliver a high dose to an area that

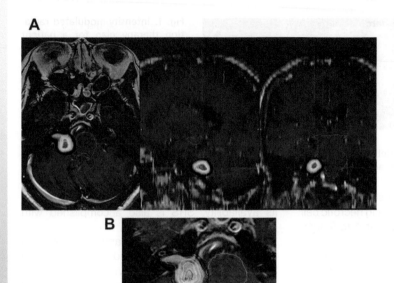

Fig. 2. (*A*) CyberKnife plan for a patient being treated for a vestibular schwannoma. She initially presented to our department with subjective hearing loss, poor word discrimination on audiometry, and some mild disequilibrium. Notice how the isodose lines compare with the plan shown in **Fig. 1**. This patient has a very high, yet inhomogeneous dose delivered to her tumor. The prescription is to 25 Gy, but, because 25 Gy is delivered to the 55% isodose line, 25 Gy is only 55% of the maximum dose within the tumor volume. Because of the physics of photons, dose falloff is sharpest near the 50% isodose line, so most SRS plans prescribe near this isodose curve. (*B*) Close-up on the target area to further define isodose curves. The brainstem, cochlea, and vestibular apparatus have been highlighted in this plan for the purposes of calculating dose to these structures. Contouring normal structures is one of the means of ensuring that dose tolerances of normal structures are not exceeded.

is readily accessible but not amenable to surgical excision. Cavities of various types fit this description.

Electrons are generally delivered only to body surfaces. They are generated with the linear accelerator by essentially removing the tungsten target from the path of the electrons. Electrons do not travel far through tissue and penetrate only deep enough to treat relatively superficial structures.

There are several reports in the literature of improved results after radiation therapy with the addition of image-guidance or MRI-based planning. For example, local control (LC) rates for meningiomas treated with radiation are excellent and seem to be improving with modern treatment techniques (MRI-based planning, strict treatment setup). Goldsmith and colleagues[5] reported that subtotally resected meningiomas treated with postoperative radiation after 1980 had better local control (LC) compared with meningiomas treated before 1980. Several more modern studies have shown excellent LC rates. For example, a series reported by Mendenhall and colleagues showed that EBRT may be equivalent to subtotal resection followed by EBRT; these investigators' 15-year LC rates exceeded 90% for both groups.[6,7]

Applications of the Delivery Methods

This article is an introduction to malignant skull base tumors. The most commonly encountered malignant skull base tumors in our practice are

atypical and malignant meningiomas. Other malignant tumors of the skull base include sinonasal undifferentiated carcinoma and soft tissue sarcomas. Chondrosarcomas and chordomas are locally aggressive, malignant tumors,.

Atypical and Malignant Meningiomas

Meningiomas are the most common benign brain tumor. Atypical and malignant meningiomas represent only a small subset: 4% to 7% and less than 5%, respectively.[8–12] Since the World Health Organization (WHO) definitions changed in 2007, many believe that the proportion of all meningiomas that are reported as atypical may have increased to as much as 25%.[13] Much of the meningioma data combines or aggregates benign, atypical, and malignant meningiomas. Because of their relative rarity, specific data on atypical and malignant meningiomas are expectedly sparse, but evolving. The following discussion extrapolates the existing data on radiotherapeutic principles and outcomes to the skull base location. **Table 2** summarizes some relevant studies.

WHEN TO TREAT: RETROSPECTIVE DATA

Although completely resected WHO grade I meningiomas do not require postoperative radiation, subtotal resection followed by adjuvant radiation achieves equivalent progression-free survival (PFS) compared with gross total resection.[7,27,28]

Table 2
Summary of relevant studies regarding adjuvant RT in the treatment of WHO II and III meningiomas

Series (Number)	Treatments	Histology	Outcomes	Comment
Adeberg et al,[14] 2012 (85)	EBRT, S + EBRT, S→EBRT	WHO II-III	II: 5-y OS 81%, 5-y PFS 50% III: 5-y OS 53%, PFS 13%	Some patients treated with carbon ion[14]
Aghi et al,[15] 2009 (108)	S (GTR), S + EBRT, S→EBRT	WHO II	5-y recurrence rate: 41% 5-y recurrence rate 0% if EBRT	No recurrences if EBRT (n = 8) 2.7 craniotomies per patient if recurrence
Attia et al,[16] 2012 (24)	SRS (salvage or primary)	WHO II	>50% OS 5 y 5-y LC 44%	Improved LC with SRS >14 Gy
Dziuk et al,[17] 1998 (27)	Primarily surgery + RT	WHO III	All: 5-y OS 57% GTR + RT: 5 y DFS 40% RT No adjuvant: 5-y DFS 16%	Benefit >60 Gy adjuvant RT ↑ recurrence interval
Goldsmith et al,[5] 1994 (23) (grade III)	Surgery + RT	WHO III	58%	>53 Gy
Goyal et al,[18] 2000 (22)	Surgery, surgery + RT in only 8 patients	WHO II	GTR: 5-y OS 87% STR: 5-y OS 100%	No benefit with RT mean dose 54 Gy
Huffman et al,[19] 2005 (21)	GKRS 18 Gy	WHO II	40% recurrence at 18–36 mo	Ref.[19]
Hug et al,[20] 2000 (16)	EBRT + S Some protons	WHO II-III	II: 5-y OS 38% III: 5-y OS 52%	Benefit with higher doses and protons
Mattozo et al,[21] 2007 (12)	SRS, EBRT	WHO I-III	II: 3-y PFS 83% III: 3-y PFS 0%	Recurrence in resection cavity common[21]
Milosevic et al,[22] 1996 (42)	Primarily surgery + RT, some surgery only	WHO II-III	5-y OS 28% 5-y CSS = 42% if >50 Gy given	Better outcome if >50 Gy Reduced LR with RT
Pasquier et al,[11] 2008 (119)	S + EBRT, S only	WHO II-III	GTR: 5-y OS 46% GTR + RT: 5-y OS 78% STR: 5-y OS 0% STR + RT: 5-y OS 56%	RT improves OS in all patients
Rosenberg and Prayson et al,[23] 2009 (13)	S + RT S + SRS	WHO III	5-y OS: 47%	Trend toward longer survival if RT given
Sughrue et al,[24,25] 2010 (63)	S + RT	WHO II-III	61% 40% at 10 y (RFS 57%, 5 y) (RFS 40%, 10 y)	Survival benefit for less extensive resection
Yang et al,[29] 2008 (33 atypical, (41 anaplastic)	S, S + EBRT	WHO II-III	II: OS atypical 11.9 y RFS atypical 11.5 y III: OS anaplastic 3.3 y RFS anaplastic 2.7 y	Adjuvant RT improved outcomes in WHO III tumors and WHO II with brain invasion
Boskos et al,[26] 2009 (24)	EBRT Protons and photons	WHO II-III	5-y OS 65% 5-y LC 61%	OS significantly associated with higher doses[26]

Data comparing specific modalities (SRS, EBRT, protons) are sparse. Data exist suggesting doses greater than 50 to 60 Gy may be ideal. None of these studies is limited to the skull base. All are retrospective, some are multi-institutional. WHO grades may be reported using different criteria (eg, 2000, 2007). The most recent change in WHO grading primarily affected the proportion of tumors classified as WHO grade II.

Abbreviations: CSS, cause-specific survival; EBRT, EBRT given at progression; GKRS, gamma knife radiosurgery; LS, local recurrence rate; OS, overall survival; PFS, progression-free survival; RFS, recurrence-free survival; S, surgery.

It is generally accepted that completely resected grade II to III should be treated with radiation postoperatively.[13,15,22,23,29] This recommendation is based on several observational studies suggesting superior outcomes (overall survival [OS], progression-free survival (PFS), LC) with adjuvant RT (eg, Refs.[17,22]). The National Comprehensive Cancer Network (NCCN) guidelines recommend that physicians consider postoperative RT for WHO grade II tumors and refer all WHO grade III tumors for postoperative RT. There are no randomized data supporting this treatment strategy and some of the data conflict with this recommendation.[18,30]

Data regarding which RT modality to choose in each situation are not extensive enough to support generation of guidelines, but experienced radiation oncologists can make this determination. Some of the data and concepts behind this reasoning are discussed.

DOSING FOR EBRT AND SRS

EBRT doses prescribed for malignant meningiomas are generally 60 Gy in 2-Gy fractions (with a 1-2 cm margin) compared with 54 Gy for benign WHO grade I meningiomas. Adjuvant or definitive SRS doses vary from 10 Gy up to 25 Gy or more but the use of radiosurgery as the primary adjuvant treatment is generally discouraged. There are some retrospective data to suggest that doses greater than 14 Gy provide superior LC for atypical meningiomas.[16] There are no randomized data to support these dose constraints, but some series have suggested that doses more than 50 Gy improve outcomes in meningiomas of all histologies (see **Table 2**).[5,20]

RECURRENCE PATTERNS INFLUENCE TREATMENT FIELDS

Recurrence patterns have been instructive in our attempt to properly define adequate dose and appropriate margins. Treating only the enhancing tumor, as is practiced with benign meningiomas, may not be the ideal strategy to control WHO grade II to III meningiomas. Of the recurrences in their series of EBRT atypical and malignant meningioma, Adeberg and colleagues[14] reported 85% of recurrences in-field, 7% at border, and 7% distant failures. (Five of these patients were treated with carbon ions, a therapy with a more restricted availability than protons, but which follows a similar physical principles.) These patients were treated with an average dose of 57.6 Gy, with a margin of 1 to 2 cm. Attia and colleagues[16] reported a series of 24 patients treated with Gamma Knife. Of the 14 recurrences, 8 recurrences were in-field,

4 at the margin, and 1 distal. Huffman and colleagues[19] also reported 21 atypical meningiomas treated with Gamma Knife, with several recurrences noted at the treatment margin but none within the field. Their prescription dose was 18 Gy. Their recurrence pattern suggests that adjacent dura should be within the SRS target. This strategy limits the applicability of SRS; irregularly shaped targets and proximity to critical structures of the skull base make extension of the target volume difficult.

Considering these data, we recommend that atypical and malignant meningiomas should receive higher doses (likely greater than or equal to 60 Gy for EBRT and greater than or equal to 14 Gy for SRS), but the dose constraints imposed by normal structures must be respected. EBRT is the preferred primary adjuvant treatment for these tumors, but SRS has and is still being used by some practitioners. A margin of 1–2 cm should be applied to malignant meningiomas. The radiation oncologist restricts and expands the margins according to anatomic barriers.

TREATMENT WITH LIMITED OR NO SURGERY

The skull base is replete with sensitive neurologic structures so gross total resections are not often feasible. It may be difficult to even perform a biopsy. Physicians are becoming increasingly comfortable treating meningiomas with RT based on imaging criteria alone. A recent series from investigators at Emory University showed that meningiomas may be treated with primary RT alone based on imaging findings. In that series, 8-year LC exceeded 90%.[31] In the absence of biopsy data, it is possible that this group contained some atypical meningiomas.

Fractionated radiation regimens typically require daily treatments for several weeks.[32] Fractionated radiation is still commonly used in the treatment of WHO grade I meningiomas in close proximity to the optic chiasm or optic nerves. This strategy is based on the observation that the EBRT can achieve effective doses for tumor control and spare function of the visual apparatus.[5,7,33] Meningiomas affecting the optic nerve sheath are exclusively treated with EBRT, with many patients reporting improved vision during treatment. No other treatment modality or combination modality has been shown to improve vision as well as RT alone for this select cohort of patients, so surgical decompression is reserved for patients with intracranial extension and rapidly evolving deficits.[34–36] Clinical symptoms and cranial nerve deficits commonly improve after radiation therapy, despite the low portion of meningiomas that recede in response to therapy.[37–40] Using these data, an atypical or malignant meningioma in this location may be treated in the same way, albeit a higher dose should be applied when possible.

Although the optic nerve may be spared with doses ranging from 50 to 54 delivered in 1.8-Gy to 2-Gy fractions, the retina and lacrimal glands may receive enough radiation to cause retinopathy or dry eyes. Also, the lens is one of the most radio-sensitive structures in the body, with doses greater than 10 Gy delivered by EBRT leading to delayed cataract formation. Thus, for optic nerve sheath meningiomas treated with fractionated RT, vision is preserved but the radiation oncologist must be attentive to potential late effects of therapy. A small British series of 34 patients showed dry eyes in 14% patients, cataracts in ~9%, and reti-nopathy in ~12% patients treated with optic nerve sheath meningiomas with radiation.[41]

Cavernous sinus and petroclival meningiomas represent an area of high surgical morbidity with extensive resection, so the use of RT is often preferred either as a primary or adjunct treatment to subtotal resection. Based on a recent literature review of cavernous sinus meningiomas treated with SRS alone, SRS results in a 3% recurrence risk, whereas subtotal resection (STR) and gross total resection (GTR) resulted in recurrence risks of 11%. Also, cranial nerve deficits were more common in the group undergoing resection.[24] One recent study involving 64 patients with cranial neuropathies showed that 53% of patients with cranial neuropathies treated within 1 year of symptom onset experienced relief compared with 26% treated more than 1 year after symptom onset, which argues for earlier therapy.[42] A second recent series published by a group in Norway showed that Gamma Knife achieved LC in 84% of patients with cavernous sinus meningioma at a median follow-up of 82 months,[43] which agrees with other data.[44,45]

PROTON THERAPY

There is a growing body of evidence supporting the use of proton radiotherapy to treat meningiomas. For example, Wenkel and colleagues[46] achieved 10-year recurrence-free rates of 88% for meningiomas treated with a combination of photons and protons, but this study was not restricted to the skull base and there were no malignant meningiomas. Also, the toxicities from treatment were slightly higher than expected for EBRT for meningiomas (1 patient death, 4 severe ophthalmologic, 4 severe neurologic, and 2 severe otologic toxicities). One report of 51 patients treated with proton SRS showed 3-year tumor control rates of 94%,

with 5.9% risk of adverse effects.[47,48] Hug and colleagues had a case series of 31 patients treated with EBRT using protons. There have been other successful studies, but preferential use of protons over conventional RT or SRS is not yet supported.

WHEN DO MENINGIOMAS RECUR?

Most meningioma recurrences after RT are noted within 2.5 years after therapy.[43,49] This situation forms the basis for close follow-up. Many centers maintain their closest follow-up within this time period (eg, MRI every 6 months for 1 year after treatment, then yearly MRI scans). A recent series of 24 patients reported by Aghi and colleagues[15] showed that atypical meningiomas fail within a similar time frame, with 7%, 41%, and 48% recurrence rates at 1, 5, and 10 years, respectively. Of the tumors treated with re-excision, only 1 of 22 transformed from atypical to malignant. Twelve of the 14 recurrences seen in a 24-patient series re-ported by Attia and colleagues[16] recurred within 2.5 years. Huffman and colleagues[19] reached a similar recurrence rate of 40% at 21 to 67 months' follow-up in their Gamma Knife series of 15 patients with atypical meningiomas.

TREATING A RECURRENCE

Atypical and malignant meningioma series show frequent recurrences after treatment with EBRT, SRS, and surgical resection. Overall, the retro-spective data seem to support decreased recur-rence risk for WHO III meningiomas treated with RT after surgery (see **Table 2**). The ideal sequence of treatment has not been established. Aghi and colleagues'[15] retrospective series showed that 53% of patients with recurrent tumors were symp-tomatic at diagnosis and reported an 86% OS rate 5 years after recurrence for atypical meningiomas. Symptoms notwithstanding, most patients are undergoing regular MRI surveillance when a recur-rence is noted.

Encouraging data exist for treatment outcomes after recurrence. Aghi and colleagues[15] reported a disease-specific survival (DSS) after recurrence of 86% at 5 years for their atypical meningioma series. Sughrue[25] reported a malignant menin-gioma series with 63 patients treated with surgery followed by adjuvant RT. There was a survival benefit observed for patients who had undergone repeat operation. Also, there was a survival benefit for STR with EBRT compared with GTR with EBRT (107 months compared with 50 months). These investigators did not observe any benefit to repeat SRS or salvage brachyther-apy after a recurrence.[25]

It seems that only a few recurrences transform into WHO grade III. Retreatments after primary therapy are common in patients with both atypical and malignant meningiomas; patients often receive multiple courses of radiation therapy (either EBRT or SRS), and may even be treated with brain brachytherapy. No guidelines exist for retreatment (or salvage therapy) based on available evidence.

SUMMARY

The heterogeneity and retrospective nature of data highlight the need for prospective clinical trials. RTOG 0539 from the Radiation Therapy Oncology Group aims to address basic management questions in meningioma patients. This trial assigns patients with low-risk meningiomas to observation. Higher-risk patients receive fractionated EBRT to 54 Gy after GTR. Patients with STR, recurrences, and WHO grade II meningiomas receive 60 Gy. EORTC 22042 trial from the European Organisation for Research and Treatment of Cancer is a phase II study in which 54 Gy is given after GTR for atypical meningiomas and 60 Gy is given malignant meningiomas or any resection extent, or atypical meningomas after STR or after recurrence. It is expected that clinical data gained from these trials will guide future treatment approaches for these common skull base tumors. At the time this article was written, data from these trials were not available.

Based on the available data, most patients with atypical meningioma can expect a prolonged disease-free interval with recurrence to be treated with a variety of modalities (see **Table 2**). Yang and colleagues[29] reported a median OS of 11.9 years in patients with atypical meningiomas and 3.3 years for anaplastic meningiomas. However, these figures were reported using WHO 2000 pathologic classification.

Chordomas and Chondrosarcomas

Chordomas are rare tumors that arise from the primitive notochord.[50] Thirty-five percent of these tumors occur at the skull base, particularly the clivus, where they invade locally. Chondrosarcomas are malignant primary bone tumors.

Chordomas invade locally and recurrence rates are high after surgery. Most recurrences are local, but many patients survive for years after recurrence. Surgery is not considered curative. There has been considerable interest in subtotal resection and adjuvant RT.

Although these tumors grow slowly, a retrospective French series showed the merits of aggressive up-front management: patients who received RT immediately after surgery versus at recurrence had a 10-year survival of 65% versus 0% for those patients treated with RT at the time of recurrence.[51] The largest series of chordomas treated with RT was conducted at Harvard University. Patients received 60 to 79.2 Cobalt-Gray-Equivalent (CGE), with LC rates at 10 years of 44%.[52,53] A recent review that pooled more than 400 patients showed that 5-year LC is nearly 70% and OS is more than 80%.[54]

RT is still associated with some morbidity: in a series reported by Noel and colleagues[55] of skull base chordomas treated with RT, hypopituitarism was seen in 25%, memory impairment in 2%, oculomotor impairment in 3%, hearing loss in 2%, and bilateral visual loss in 2%.

Chondrosarcomas are a group of different sarcomas that commonly occur at the skull base. Because of their rarity and presentation, which are similar to chordomas, chordomas are often grouped along with chondrosarcomas for retrospective and prospective series. For example, Hug and colleagues[56] studied adjuvant proton beam EBRT after resection for chordomas and chondrosarcomas. Five-year LC and OS exceeded 90%, better than LC and OS seen in chordomas. Studies from MGH concurred with this finding.[57,58]

Adjuvant therapy with chondrosarcomas and chordomas is largely accomplished with proton EBRT. Protons are particularly useful in these tumors: they may encompass an area too large for SRS, and achieve a high enough dose with generally acceptable toxicity that is not otherwise achievable with EBRT. However, advanced treatment planning technologies are able to compensate for the less favorable dose distribution traditionally achieved with conventional EBRT techniques. Some practitioners are increasingly using sophisticated planning strategies to treat these tumors and improve access for patients who otherwise may not be able to afford logistics costs of a proton treatment at a distant center.

Other Sarcomas of the Head and Neck

Soft tissue sarcomas of the skull base are usually treated maximal surgical excision, followed by post-operative radiation therapy. Recurrence risk is higher than soft tissue sarcomas of the extremities, because clean surgical margins cannot often be achieved. The techniques applied to other soft tissue sarcomas of the head and neck include: EBRT, SRS, intraoperative RT, and brachytherapy. Specific data on skull base sarcomas are even more limited than the other entities discussed in this article, and no clear treatment standard is defined.

Sinonasal Carcinoma

The sinonasal cavities present the surgeon with a difficult anatomic location, which often precludes safe debulking and clear margins. RT is critical in these tumors. The high doses of radiation necessary for controlling these tumors are often limited by the adjacent critical structures (optic nerves, oropharynx, brain parenchyma, eye, and retina). Orbital invasion and invasion through the cribriform plate necessitate a multidisciplinary approach involving neurosurgeons and head and neck surgeons. This is an extraordinarily rare tumor, so data are sparse.

INDICATIONS FOR RT

RT may be given to the tumor bed after resection or it may be used for primary treatment along with chemotherapy in unresectable tumors.[58]

RT TECHNIQUES

The sinonasal carcinomas are an ideal example to discuss advances in treatment planning. In the early days of radiation therapy, anteroposterior/posteroanterior fields were common for all body sites. Modern EBRT delivered to sensitive sites uses three-dimensional conformal RT (3D-CRT) and intensity modulated radiation therapy (IMRT). 3D-CRT delivers radiation usually in a coplanar fashion, but from multiple beam angles like spokes on a wheel. IMRT is the technique that allows beam energies to vary at different beam positions. This technique has significantly advanced our ability to treat tumors in sensitive locations.

Hoppe and colleagues found a lower than expected incidence of grade 3 toxicities in their series with a 5 yr OS of 67%, survival comparable to other published series but with lesser observed toxicity.[59–62]

In a study by Monroe and colleagues[63] focusing on radiation retinopathy, hyperfractionation (2 smaller doses delivered per day) resulted in lower rates of radiation-induced retinopathy, even when total doses were comparable. The series included 168 patients, 64 of whom had paranasal sinus tumors. Recall that normal tissue recovers from radiation with time, so dividing the dose into smaller fractions should logically spare normally functioning tissues to a greater degree and this study seems to support this.

REFERENCES

1. Levin WP, Kooy H, Loeffler JS, et al. Proton beam therapy. Br J Cancer 2005;93:849–54.

2. Debus J, Wuendrich M, Pirzkall A, et al. High efficacy of fractionated stereotactic radiotherapy of large base of skull meningiomas: long term results. J Clin Oncol 2001;19(15):3547–53.

3. Meijer OW, Weijmans EJ, Knol DL, et al. Tumor volume changes after radiosurgery for vestibular schwannoma: implications for follow up MR imaging protocol. AJNR Am J Neuroradiol 2008;29(5):906–10.

4. Kollova A, Liscak R, Novotny J, et al. Gamma Knife surgery for benign meningioma. J Neurosurg 2007;107(2):325–36.

5. Goldsmith BJ, Wara WM, Wilson CB, et al. Postoperative irradiation for subtotally resected meningiomas: a retrospective analysis of 140 patients treated from 1967 to 1990. J Neurosurg 1994;80(2):195–201.

6. Mendenhall WM, Morris CG, Amdur RJ, et al. Radiotherapy alone or after subtotal resection for benign skull base meningiomas. Cancer 2003;98(7):1473.

7. Glaholm J, Bloom HJ, Crow JH, et al. The role of radiotherapy in the management of intracranial meningiomas: the Royal Marsden Hospital experience with 186 patients. Int J Radiat Oncol Biol Phys 1990;18:755–61.

8. Whittle IR, Smith C, Navoo P, et al. Meningiomas. Lancet 2004;363:1535–43.

9. Kleihues P, Burger PC, Scheithauer BW. Histologic typing of tumors of the central nervous system. 2nd edition. Berlin: Springer-Verlag; 1993.

10. Kleihues P, Cavenee WK. Pathology and genetics of tumors of the nervous system. 2nd edition. Lyon (France): IARC Press; 2000.

11. Pasquier D, Bijmolt S, Veninga T, et al. Atypical and malignant meningioma: outcome and prognostic factors in 119 irradiated patients. A multicenter, retrospective study of the rare cancer network. Int J Radiat Oncol Biol Phys 2008;71:1388–93.

12. Mahmood A, Caccamo DV, Tomecek FJ, et al. Atypical and malignant meningiomas: a clinicopathological review. Neurosurgery 1993;33:955–63.

13. Hanft S, Canoll P, Bruce JN. A review of malignant meningiomas: diagnosis, characteristics, and treatment. J Neurooncol 2010;99:433–43.

14. Adeberg S, Hartmann C, Welzel T, et al. Long-term outcome after radiotherapy in patients with atypical and malignant meningiomas–clinical results in 85 patients treated in a single institution leading to optimized guidelines for early radiation therapy. Int J Radiat Oncol Biol Phys 2012;83(3):859–64.

15. Aghi MK, Carter BS, Cosgrove GR, et al. Long-term recurrence rates of atypical meningiomas after gross total resection with or without postoperative adjuvant radiation. Neurosurgery 2009;64(1):56–60.

16. Attia A, Chan MD, Mott RT. Patterns of failure after treatment of atypical meningioma with gamma knife radiosurgery. J Neurooncol 2012;108(1):179–85.

17. Dziuk TW, Woo S, Butler EB, et al. Malignant meningioma: an indication for initial aggressive surgery

and adjuvant radiotherapy. J Neurooncol 1998; 37(2):177.

18. Goyal LK, Suh JH, Mohan DS, et al. Local control and overall survival in atypical meningioma: a retrospective study. Int J Radiat Oncol Biol Phys 2000; 46(1):57–61.

19. Huffman BC, Reinacher PC, Gilbach JM. Gamma knife surgery for atypical meningiomas. J Neurosurg 2005;102(Suppl):283.

20. Hug EB, Devries A, Thornton AF, et al. Management of atypical and malignant meningiomas: role of high-dose, 3D-conformal radiation therapy. J Neurooncol 2000;48:151–60.

21. Mattozo CA, De Salles AA, Klement IA. Stereotactic radiation treatment for recurrent nonbenign meningiomas. J Neurosurg 2007;106(5):846–54.

22. Milosevic MF, Frost PJ, Laperriere NJ, et al. Radiotherapy for atypical or malignant intracranial meningioma. Int J Radiat Oncol Biol Phys 1996;34(4):817–22.

23. Rosenberg LS, Prayson RA, Lee J, et al. Long-term experience with World Health Organization grade III (malignant) meningiomas at a single institution. Int J Radiat Oncol Biol Phys 2009;74(2):427.

24. Sughrue ME, Rutkowski MJ, Aranda D, et al. Factors affecting outcome following treatment of patients with cavernous sinus meningiomas. J Neurosurg 2010;113(5):1087–92.

25. Sughrue ME, Sanai N, Shangari G, et al. Outcome and survival following primary and repeat surgery for World Health Organization Grade III meningiomas. J Neurosurg 2010;113(2):202.

26. Boskos C, Feuvret L, Noel G, et al. Combined proton and photon conformal radiotherapy for intracranial atypical and malignant meningioma. Int J Radiat Oncol Biol Phys 2009;75(2):399.

27. Forbes AR, Goldberg ID. Radiation therapy in the treatment of meningioma: the Joint Center for Radiation Therapy experience 1970 to 1982. J Clin Oncol 1984;2(10):1139.

28. Taylor BW Jr, Marcus RB Jr, Friedman WA, et al. The meningioma controversy: postoperative radiation therapy. Int J Radiat Oncol Biol Phys 1988;15(2):299.

29. Yang SY, Park CK, Park SH, et al. Atypical and anaplastic meningiomas: prognostic implications of clinicopathologic features. J Neurol Neurosurg Psychiatry 2008;79:574–80.

30. Stessin AM, Schwartz A, Judanin G, et al. Does adjuvant external-beam radiotherapy improve outcomes for nonbenign meningiomas? A Surveillance, Epidemiology, and End Results (SEER)-based analysis. J Neurosurg 2012.

31. Korah MP, Nowlan AW, Johnstone PA, et al. Radiation therapy alone for imaging-defined meningiomas. Int J Radiat Oncol Biol Phys 2010;76(1):181.

32. Uy NW, Woo SY, The BS, et al. Intensity-modulated radiation therapy (IMRT) for meningioma. Int J Radiat Oncol Biol Phys 2002;53:1265–70.

33. Miralbell R, Linggood RM, de la Monte S, et al. The role of radiotherapy in the treatment of subtotally resected benign meningiomas. J Neurooncol 1992; 13:157–64.

34. Turbin RE, Thompson CR, Kennerdell JS, et al. A long-term visual outcome comparison in patients with optic nerve sheath meningioma managed with observation, surgery, radiotherapy, or surgery and radiotherapy. Ophthalmology 2002;109(5):890.

35. Rogers CL. Radiation therapy for intracranial meningiomas. In: Mehta MP, editor. Principles and practice of neuro-oncology: a multi-disciplinary approach. New York: Demos Medical; 2011. p. 820–41.

36. Roser F, Nakamura M, Martini-Thomas R, et al. The role of surgery in meningiomas involving the optic nerve sheath. Clin Neurol Neurosurg 2006;108(5):470–6.

37. Litre CF, Colin P, Noudel R, et al. Fractionated stereotactic radiotherapy treatment of cavernous sinus meningiomas: a study of 100 cases. Int J Radiat Oncol Biol Phys 2009;74(4):1012–7.

38. Henzel M, Gross MW, Hamm K, et al. Stereotactic radiotherapy of meningiomas: symptomatology, acute and late toxicity. Strahlenther Onkol 2006; 182(7):382–8.

39. Milker-Zabel S, Zabel A, Schulz-Ertner D, et al. Fractionated stereotactic radiotherapy in patients with benign or atypical intracranial meningioma: long-term experience and prognostic factors. Int J Radiat Oncol Biol Phys 2005;61(3):809–16.

40. Noel G, Bollet MA, Calugaru V, et al. Functional outcome of patients with benign meningioma treated by 3D conformal irradiation with a combination of photons and protons. Int J Radiat Oncol Biol Phys 2005;62(5):1412–22.

41. Saeed P, Blank L, Selva D, et al. Primary radiotherapy in progressive optic nerve sheath meningiomas: a long term follow up study. Br J Ophthalmol 2010; 94(5):564.

42. Spiegelman R, Cohen ZR, Nissim O, et al. Cavernous sinus meningiomas: a large LINAC radiosurgery series. J Neurooncol 2010;98(2):195.

43. Skeie BS, Enger PO, Dkeie GO, et al. Gamma knife surgery of meningiomas involving the cavernous sinus: long term follow up of 100 patients. Neurosurgery 2010;66(4):661.

44. Lee JY, Niranjan A, McInerney J, et al. Stereotactic radiosurgery providing long-term tumor control of cavernous sinus meningiomas. J Neurosurg 2002;97(1):65.

45. Nicolato A, Foroni R, Alessandrini F, et al. Radiosurgical treatment of cavernous sinus meningiomas: experience with 122 treated patients. Neurosurgery 2002;51(5):1153.

46. Wenkel E, Thornton AF, Finkelstein D, et al. Benign meningioma: partially resected, biopsied, and recurrent intracranial tumors treated with combined proton and photon radiotherapy. Int J Radiat Oncol Biol Phys 2000;48(5):1363–70.

47. Halasz LM, Bussiere MR, Dennies ER, et al. Proton stereotactic radiosurgery for the treatment of benign meningiomas. Int J Radiat Oncol Biol Phys 2011; 81(5):1428.

48. Goldsmith BJ, Rosenthal SA, Wara WM, et al. Optic neuropathy after irradiation of meningioma. Radiology 1992;185:71–6.

49. Pirzkall A, Debus J, Haering P, et al. Intensity modulated radiotherapy (IMRT) for recurrent, residual, or untreated skull-base meningiomas: preliminary clinical experience. Int J Radiat Oncol Biol Phys 2003; 55:362–72.

50. McMaster ML, Goldstein AM, Bromley CM, et al. Chordoma: incidence and survival patterns in the United States, 1973-1995. Cancer Causes Control 2001;12:1–11.

51. Carpentier A, Polivka M, Blanquet A, et al. Suboccipital and cervical chordomas: the value of aggressive treatment at first presentation of disease. J Neurosurg 2002;97:1070–7.

52. Debus J, Hug EB, Liebsch NJ, et al. Brainstem tolerance to conformal radiotherapy of skull base tumors. Int J Radiat Oncol Biol Phys 1997;39(5): 967–75.

53. Terahara A, Niemierko A, Goitein M, et al. Analysis of the relationship between tumor dose inhomogeneity and local control in patients with skull base chordoma. Int J Radiat Oncol Biol Phys 1999;45:351–8.

54. Amichetti M, Cianchetti M, Amelio D, et al. Proton therapy in chordomas of the base of the skull: a systematic review. Neurosurg Rev 2009; 32(4):403.

55. Noel G, Habrand JL, Jauffret E, et al. Radiation therapy for chordoma and chondrosarcoma of the skull base and the cervical spine. Prognostic factors and patterns of failure. Strahlenther Onkol 2003;179: 241–8.

56. Hug EB, Loredo LN, Slater JD, et al. Proton radiation therapy for chordomas and chondrosarcomas of the skull base. J Neurosurg 1999;91(3):432–9.

57. Rosenberg AE, Nielsen GP, Keel SB, et al. Chondrosarcoma of the base of the skull: a clinicopathologic study of 200 cases with emphasis on its distinction from chordoma. Am J Surg Pathol 1999;23(11): 1370–8.

58. Robbins KT, Ferlito A, Silver CE, et al. Contemporary management of sinonasal cancer. Head Neck 2011; 33(9):1352.

59. Duthoy W, Boterberg T, Claus F, et al. Postoperative intensity-modulated radiotherapy in sinonasal carcinoma. Cancer 2005;104(1):71–82.

60. Chen AM, Daly ME, El-Sayed I. Patterns of failure after combined-modality approaches incorporating radiotherapy for sinonasal undifferentiated carcinoma of the head and neck. Int J Radiat Oncol Biol Phys 2008;70(2):338–43.

61. Al-Mamgani A, van Rooij P, Mehilal R, et al. Combined-modality treatment improved outcomes in sinonasal undifferentiated carcinoma: single-institutional experience of 21 patients and review of the literature. Eur Arch Otorhinolaryngol 2012. [Epub ahead of print].

62. Hoppe BS, Stegman LD, Zelefsky MJ, et al. Treatment of nasal cavity and paranasal sinus cancer with modern radiotherapy techniques in the postoperative setting–the MSKCC experience. Int J Radiat Oncol Biol Phys 2007;67(3):691.

63. Monroe AT, Bhandare N, Morris CG, et al. Preventing radiation retinopathy with hyperfractionation. Int J Radiat Oncol Biol Phys 2005;61(3):856–64.

Index

Note: Page numbers of article titles are in **boldface** type.

Neurosurg Clin N Am 24 (2013) 137–142
http://dx.doi.org/10.1016/S1042-3680(12)00126-X

Moving?

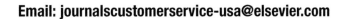

Make sure your subscription moves with you!

To notify us of your new address, find your **Clinics Account Number** (located on your mailing label above your name), and contact customer service at:

Email: journalscustomerservice-usa@elsevier.com

800-654-2452 (subscribers in the U.S. & Canada)
314-447-8871 (subscribers outside of the U.S. & Canada)

Fax number: 314-447-8029

Elsevier Health Sciences Division
Subscription Customer Service
3251 Riverport Lane
Maryland Heights, MO 63043

ELSEVIER

Printed and bound by CPI Group (UK) Ltd, Croydon, CR0 4YY

03/10/2024

01040347-0007